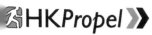 **HKPropel** 》 Accessing your HK*Propel* digital product is e

T0260480

INSTRUCTORS: Use the access instructions provided by your sales rep. inste
student access code below.

If it's your first time using HK*Propel*:

1. Visit HKPropel.HumanKinetics.com.
2. Click the "New user? Register here" link on the opening screen to register for an account and redeem your one-time-use access code.
3. Follow the onscreen prompts to create your HK*Propel* account. Use a **valid email address** as your username to ensure you receive important system updates and to help us find your account if you ever need assistance.
4. Enter the access code exactly as shown below, including hyphens. You will not need to re-enter this access code on subsequent visits, and this access code cannot be redeemed by any other user.
5. After your first visit, simply log in to HKPropel.HumanKinetics.com to access your digital product.

If you already have an HK*Propel* account:

1. Visit HKPropel.HumanKinetics.com and log in with your username (email address) and password.
2. Once you are logged in, click the arrow next to your name in the top right corner and then click **My Account**.
3. Under the "Add Access Code" heading, enter the access code exactly as shown below, including hyphens, and click the **Add** button.
4. Once your code is redeemed, navigate to your Library on the Dashboard to access your digital content.

Product: Applied Biomechanics Laboratory Manual HKPropel Online Video

Student access code: TDDX-OCEA-ZCV3-C8TC

NOTE TO STUDENTS: If your instructor uses HK*Propel* to assign work to your class, you will need to enter a **class enrollment token** in HK*Propel* on the **My Account** page. This token will be provided **by your instructor at no cost to you**, but it is required **in addition** to the unique access code that is printed above.

Helpful tips:

You may reset your password from the log in screen at any time if you forget it.

Your license to this digital product will expire **2 years** after the date you redeem the access code. You can check the expiration dates of all your HK*Propel* products at any time in **My Account**.

For assistance, contact us via email at HKPropelCustSer@hkusa.com.   04-2022

Applied Biomechanics Laboratory Manual

John C. Garner, PhD
Troy University

Charles R. Allen, PhD
Florida Southern College

Harish Chander, PhD
Mississippi State University

Adam C. Knight, PhD
Mississippi State University

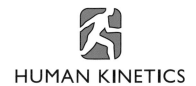

HUMAN KINETICS

Library of Congress Cataloging-in-Publication Data

Names: Garner, John C., III, 1979- author.
Title: Applied biomechanics laboratory manual / John C. Garner, III,
 Charles Allen, Harish Chander, Adam C Knight.
Description: Champaign, IL : Human Kinetics, [2023] | Includes
 bibliographical references and index.
Identifiers: LCCN 2022001895 (print) | LCCN 2022001896 (ebook) | ISBN
 9781718207417 (spiral bound) | ISBN 9781718207424 (epub) | ISBN
 9781718207431 (pdf)
Subjects: LCSH: Human mechanics--Laboratory manuals. |
 Biomechanics--Laboratory manuals. | BISAC: MEDICAL / Physical Medicine &
 Rehabilitation | MEDICAL / Orthopedics
Classification: LCC QP303 .G37 2023 (print) | LCC QP303 (ebook) | DDC
 612.7/6--dc23/eng/20220309
LC record available at https://lccn.loc.gov/2022001895
LC ebook record available at https://lccn.loc.gov/2022001896

ISBN: 978-1-7182-0741-7 (loose-leaf)

Copyright © 2023 by Human Kinetics, Inc.

Acquisitions Editor: Jolynn Gower; **Developmental Editor:** Melissa J. Zavala; **Copyeditor:** Janet Kiefer; **Proofreader:** James Barnett; **Permissions Manager:** Dalene Reeder; **Graphic Designer:** Denise Lowry; **Cover Designer:** Keri Evans; **Cover Design Specialist:** Susan Rothermel Allen; **Photograph (cover):** © microgen / iStock/Getty Images; **Photographer:** Gregg Henness; **Photographs (interior):** © Human Kinetics, unless otherwise noted; **Photo Production Specialist:** Amy M. Rose; **Photo Production Manager:** Jason Allen; **Senior Art Manager:** Kelly Hendren; **Illustrations:** © Human Kinetics, unless otherwise noted; **Printer:** Walsworth

We thank Mississippi State University for assistance in providing the location for the photo and video shoot for this book.

Printed in the United States of America   10 9 8 7 6 5 4 3 2 1

The paper in this book was manufactured using responsible forestry methods.

Human Kinetics
1607 N. Market Street
Champaign, IL 61820
USA

United States and International
Website: **US.HumanKinetics.com**
Email: info@hkusa.com
Phone: 1-800-747-4457

Canada
Website: **Canada.HumanKinetics.com**
Email: info@hkcanada.com

E8355 (loose-leaf)

Tell us what you think!
Human Kinetics would love to hear what we can do to improve the customer experience. Use this QR code to take our brief survey.

CONTENTS

LABORATORY ACTIVITY FINDER

PREFACE

Focused on foundational information, *Applied Biomechanics Laboratory Manual* offers students and instructors a practical application of fundamental topics within the field of biomechanics. With 13 easy-to-follow labs that focus on foundational information, readers will gain applied biomechanical knowledge and skills to use in fields of allied health, sports performance, and ergonomics.

Applied Biomechanics Laboratory Manual is organized into three major sections covering basic kinesiological terminology and movement descriptions, fundamental biomechanical principles, and applied biomechanics for the practitioner. Students and instructors will be able to apply the fundamental theoretical information gleaned from lecture-based courses in a simple, yet complete model of laboratory exercises.

The progression of labs through the increasingly in-depth material, along with easy-to-follow instructions, forms, and worksheets make this lab manual an excellent experiential component for a course in biomechanics. Each lab features the same straightforward format outlining the purpose of the lab, materials required, background information, procedures, assignments, and references. Related online learning tools delivered through HK *Propel* include digital versions of the forms found in the book as well as online video clips that simulate the experience of performing many of the lab activities.

The authors have carefully designed the laboratories to use relatively inexpensive and readily available materials in an academic kinesiology or exercise science program. Further, these labs have been thoroughly tested through many years of instruction by students with a wide variety of talents and interests. Our students have enjoyed their experiences using these laboratory exercises and we hope yours will, too.

Movement Terminology

Objectives

- Understand the definitions and terminologies associated with describing human movement.
- Understand the terminology for describing body part locations, reference positions, and anatomical orientations.
- Demonstrate joint movements and muscle actions individually and in real-life situations.

DEFINITIONS

Anatomical Directional Terminologies

anterior—A position closer to the front of the body than another structure is.

deep—A position closer to the inside of the body than another structure is.

distal—A position farther from the midline than another structure is.

dorsal—The top of the foot or the back of the hand.

inferior—A position lower in the vertical direction than another structure.

palmar and plantar—The bottom of the palm and foot, respectively.

posterior—A position closer to the back of the body than another structure is.

proximal—A position closer to the midline than another structure is.

superficial—A position closer to the surface of the body than another structure is.

superior—A position higher in the vertical direction than another structure is.

Muscle and Joint Terminologies

active range of motion—A joint action that is performed by the muscles that cross that joint.

agonist—The muscle most responsible for the joint action.

antagonist—The muscle that performs the opposite joint action of the agonist.

fixators—The muscles that help stabilize the proximal joints in relation to the joint being moved.

insertion—The attachment site of a muscle that does move. In the past it has been referred to the *distal attachment*.

origin—The attachment site of a muscle that does not move. In the past it has been referred to the *proximal attachment*.

passive ROM—A joint action that is performed without intrinsic muscle activity.

range of motion (ROM)—The angular distance through which a joint can be moved, either actively or passively.

resistive ROM—Joint action performed against an external resistance.

synergist—The muscles that help or aid the prime movers.

Biomechanics is the science concerned with the internal and external forces acting on the human body and the effects produced by these forces. (The prefix *bio* means living or biological systems, and the word root *mechanics* means analysis of forces and their effects.) Biomechanics is also commonly described as the application of mechanical principles to the study of biological systems. Kinesiology is defined as the study of anatomy, physiology, and mechanics as it pertains to human movement. Understanding medical terms associated with biomechanics and kinesiology is beneficial for health care professionals and health-related professionals such as physicians, physician assistants, physical therapists and physical therapy assistants, occupational therapists and occupational therapy assistants, athletic trainers, strength and conditioning coaches, exercise physiologists, biomechanists, and physical educators.

ANATOMIC NEUTRAL POSITION

Anatomic neutral is the reference position of the human body. It consists of the body standing erect with face and chin straight, earlobes level, shoulders level, arms at the sides, palms facing forward, equal spacing between both elbows and the trunk, feet facing forward, and toes pointed slightly outward (figure 1.1). This position is the same even if the individual is lying down. It is from this position that each movement is described and from which the normal and abnormal ranges of motion (ROM) are

calculated. It is also seen as the starting point in describing the range of motion at all joints. Anatomic fundamental neutral is the same position but with the arms rotated medially. This medial rotation occurs at the glenohumeral joint. The movements of the forearm can be described from the fundamental position, and it denotes the normal stance of an individual and from where the activities of daily living are performed.

PLANES AND AXES

Planes are slices in space that continue infinitely in all directions. With regard to anatomy, planes divide the body into panels within which movement occurs. The real power of anatomical planes is that they unify the language that is used to describe a movement to someone who may not be able to see the movement being performed. The three anatomical are the sagittal, frontal, and transverse planes (figure 1.2).

Sagittal Plane

The sagittal plane is the vertical plane that divides the body into right and left parts. Move-

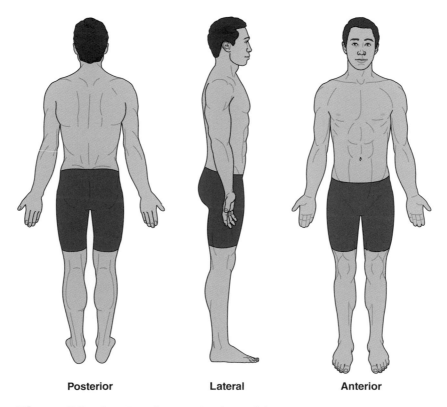

Posterior   Lateral   Anterior

Figure 1.1 Anatomic neutral position.

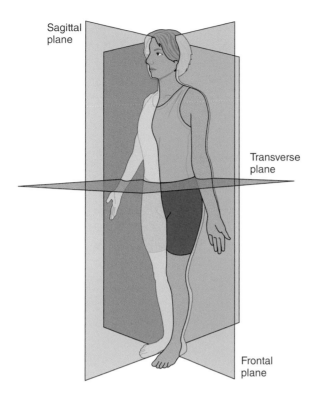

Sagittal plane

Transverse plane

Frontal plane

Figure 1.2   Sagittal, frontal, and transverse planes.

ment occurs about the mediolateral axis. Flexion and extension movements commonly occur in this plane.

Frontal Plane

The frontal plane is the vertical plane that divides the body into anterior and posterior parts. Movements occur about the anterior and posterior axes. Abduction and adduction movements commonly occur in this plane.

Transverse Plane

The transverse plane is the horizontal plane that divides the body into inferior and superior parts. Movements occur about the polar or vertical axis. Rotation movements commonly occur in this plane.

Diagonal Planes of Motion

Diagonal planes of motion are where movements occur in a combination of joints and planes. Our activities of daily living often occur in this type of plane. The upper body has a high diagonal plane of motion and a low diagonal plane of motion.

The upper body, high diagonal plane is used for overhand movements or overhead skills of the upper limbs at the shoulder joints (e.g., cricket bowling, baseball pitching). The upper body, low diagonal plane is used for underhand skills of the upper limbs at shoulder joints (e.g., snow bowling, softball pitching). Finally, the lower body, low diagonal plane is used for movements of the lower limbs at the hip joints (e.g., soccer kicks).

Joint Actions

Synovial or freely movable joints, based on a structural classification, can be of different types and move in different number of planes about their corresponding axis. A list of basic joint types and their number of planes of movement about their corresponding axis is provided in table 1.1.

Table 1.1   Joint Types and Number of Planes of Movement

Joints	Axis	Plane
Hinge	1	1
Pivot	1	1
Condyloid	2	2
Ellipsoid	2	2
Saddle	3	3
Ball and socket	3	3

Flexion—These joint motions move the segments in such a manner as to roll them up. It typically causes a decrease in the angle between two segments. Overall, these joint motions will bring the segments closer to a position that mimics the fetal position.

Extension—These joint motions move the segments in such a manner as to unroll them. It typically causes an increase in the angle between two segments. Overall, these joint motions will bring the segments back from a fetal position and closer to an anatomical position.

Abduction—The limb segment is moved away from the midline of the body.

Adduction—The limb segment is moved toward the midline of the body.

Internal rotation—The limb segment is rotated about its long axis with the anterior surface moving toward the midline of the body.

External rotation—The limb segment is rotated about its long axis with the anterior surface moving away the midline of the body.

Special Joint Action Names

Ankle

Dorsiflexion—Action in which the distance between the top of the foot and the anterior surface of the lower leg is decreased.

Plantar flexion—Action in which the distance between the top of the foot and the anterior surface of the lower leg is increased.

Inversion—Action in which the big toe is moved upward and toward the midline of the body (this is the classic ankle sprain posture).

Eversion—Action in which the big toe is moved downward and away from the midline of the body.

Hip or Shoulder

Horizontal abduction—With the limb segment flexed, it is moved in the transverse plane, away from the midline.

Horizontal adduction—With the limb segment flexed, it is moved in the transverse plane, toward the midline.

Circumduction—This is a combination movement that includes flexion, extension, abduction, and adduction of the limb. In this motion, the segment sweeps out a cone, in a multiplanar motion. (Note: There is no rotation associated with this motion.)

Shoulder Girdle (Scapula)

These motions are described by the motion of the entire of scapula.

Upward rotation—The inferior angle moves upward and laterally.

Downward rotation—The inferior angle moves downward and medially.

Protraction (abduction)—The vertebral border of the scapula moves away from the midline (spine).

Retraction (adduction)—The vertebral border of the scapula moves toward the midline (spine).

Elevation—The scapula moves upward.

Depression—The scapula moves downward.

Radioulnar Joint

Pronation—This joint position can be identified by the thumb location. When the thumb is positioned on the medial side of the elbow, the radioulnar joint is in pronation.

Supination—This joint position can be identified by the thumb location. When the thumb is positioned on the lateral side of the elbow, the radioulnar joint is in supination.

Wrist

Radial deviation—Action in which the angle between the thumb and the radius decreases.

Ulna deviation—Action in which the angle between the pinky and the ulna decreases.

Muscle Actions

A muscle action is brought about when tension or force is developed in a muscle. Muscle actions can cause, control, or prevent joint movement depending on the type of action. All muscle actions are either isometric or isotonic. Isometric can be described as a static muscle action, while isotonic can be described as a dynamic muscle action. Isometric and isotonic dynamic muscle actions can further be classified as either concentric or eccentric.

Hence, we will discuss the three important true muscle actions:

1. **Concentric**—Muscle action in which the muscle shortens under tension.
2. **Eccentric**—Muscle action in which the muscle lengthens under tension.
3. **Isometric**—Muscle action in which the length of the muscle remains the same under tension.

We will focus on these three muscle actions. However, the reader should be aware that there are three externally controlled muscle actions as well, which are primarily used in rehabilitation:

- **Isokinetic**—Muscle action in which the length of the muscle changes at the same speed throughout the range of motion (same speed, variable resistance).

- **Isotonic**—Muscle action in which the tension of the muscle remains the same throughout the entire range of motion (variable speed, same resistance).

- **Isoinertial**—Muscle action in which the external load remains the same throughout the entire range of motion.

Movement Analysis of Specific Tasks

Equipment

- Dumbbells
- Group laboratory report

Biceps Curl

In this laboratory activity, you will utilize your knowledge of human movement to fill in the cells in the laboratory activity tables on the group laboratory report by placing the correct joint action with the corresponding plane and axis. As a class, every student will take turns in demonstrating joint actions, while the others will record the joint actions.

Step 1:   Choose a student volunteer.

Step 2:   Have the volunteer stand in an anatomical neutral position holding a dumbbell of their choice unilaterally (one arm) or bilaterally (both arms).

Step 3:   Instruct the volunteer to perform a normal paced movement of the upward phase of a biceps curl exercise followed by returning back to the starting position (downward phase).

Step 4:   Have the class record the joint action in the appropriate cells on the group laboratory report.

LABORATORY ACTIVITY 1.1

GROUP LABORATORY REPORT

Laboratory Activity 1.1 Table 1 Biceps Curl Upward (Concentric) Phase

Joint (movement)	Start position	Joint action or actions	Plane	Axis
Scapula				
Glenohumeral				
Elbow				
Radioulnar				
Hip				
Knee				
Ankle				

Laboratory Activity 1.1 Table 2 Biceps Curl Downward (Eccentric) Phase

Joint (movement)	Start position	Joint action or actions	Plane	Axis
Scapula				
Glenohumeral				
Elbow				
Radioulnar				
Hip				
Knee				
Ankle				

From J. Garner, C. Allen, H. Chander, and A. Knight, *Applied Biomechanics Laboratory Manual*. (Champaign, IL: Human Kinetics, 2023).

Movement Analysis of Specific Tasks

Equipment

- Completed group laboratory report
- Individual laboratory report

Squat Jump With Arm Swing

In this lab activity, you will use the information in laboratory activity tables 1.1 and 1.2 to analyze movements. To complete this task, you will work in groups of two. One member of your group will act out the movement while the other student fills in the appropriate cells in the laboratory activity 1.2 tables on the individual laboratory report. You will switch roles after completing the first movement.

Step 1: Decide who will perform the exercise first.

Step 2: Have the volunteer stand in an anatomical neutral position.

Step 3: Instruct the volunteer to perform a normal paced movement of a downward phase of squat until the upper leg is parallel to the floor and then propel upward in a jumping motion using both arms in a swinging motion.

Step 4: Tell the volunteer to attempt to land with both feet and then return to starting position for both upper and lower extremities.

Step 5: Record your findings in the individual laboratory report.

Question Set 1.1 and 1.2

1. Complete the following directional terminology questions:

    a. In anatomical position, the wrist joint is more _____ compared to the shoulder joint.

    b. In anatomical position with reference to the shoulder joint, the wrist joint is more _____ compared to the elbow joint.

    c. In anatomical position, the head is more _____ compared to the sternum.

2. Perform sagittal plane movements of the joints listed next in active full range of motion and arrange them from least total range of motion to most total range of motion.

    a. Ankle

    b. Knee

    c. Hip

    d. Wrist

    e. Elbow

    f. Shoulder

3. Which of the following movements have a greater ROM compared to the other? Also provide a rationale for the difference in ROM.
   a. Ankle inversion versus eversion
   b. Wrist radial deviation versus ulnar deviation
   c. Hip flexion versus extension
4. Create tables like the laboratory activity tables of the lab to fill out for the following exercise phases.
   a. Seated row (pulling or concentric phase)
   b. Seated row (eccentric phase)
   c. Barbell reverse lunge (downward or eccentric phase)—right side when left side goes back
   d. Barbell reverse lunge (upward or concentric phase)—right side when left side goes back
   e. Lateral pull-down (pulling or concentric phase)
   f. Lateral pull-down (eccentric phase)

LABORATORY ACTIVITY 1.2

INDIVIDUAL LABORATORY REPORT

Participant name or ID number: _____ Date: _____

Tester: _____ Time: _____

Participant age: _____ Height: _____ Weight: _____ Sex: _____

Laboratory Activity 1.2 Table 1   Squat Jump With Arm Swing Downward Phase

Joint (movement)	Start position	Joint action or actions	Plane	Axis
Scapula				
Glenohumeral				
Elbow				
Radioulnar				
Hip				
Knee				
Ankle				

Laboratory Activity 1.2 Table 2   Squat Jump With Arm Swing Upward Phase

Joint (movement)	Start position	Joint action or actions	Plane	Axis
Scapula				
Glenohumeral				
Elbow				
Radioulnar				
Hip				
Knee				
Ankle				

From J. Garner, C. Allen, H. Chander, and A. Knight, *Applied Biomechanics Laboratory Manual*. (Champaign, IL: Human Kinetics, 2023).

Goniometry and Anthropometry

Objectives

- Understand the principles of range of motion (ROM) of a synovial (freely movable) joint.
- Understand the differences in active and passive ROM and measurement of the ROM using a goniometer.
- Learn to measure active and passive ROM of major upper extremity and lower extremity joints.
- Understand principles of body segment shapes and sizes.
- Learn to measure body segments using Dempster's anthropometry data (Dempster, 1955).

DEFINITIONS

anthropometry—The science of measuring an individual's size, form, and physical features, which include body weight, height, skinfold thickness, body segment circumferences, and body segment lengths.

end feel—The sensation experienced by the examiner performing passive range of motion movements at the end of the range of a joint. It can also be thought of as the resistance to range of motion at the end range of the joint, denoting the maximum range of motion available at that joint, especially when measuring using a goniometer. End feels can be of various types, such as capsular, ligamentous, bony, soft tissue approximation, muscle stretch, and empty (pain).

goniometry—Derived from the Greek words *gonia*, meaning angle, and *metron*, meaning measurement; the science of measuring a joint's range of motion or its position using a device called a goniometer, which has three distinct parts: a body with a central axis, a stationary arm, and a moving arm.

range of motion (ROM)—The range in which a joint can be moved freely and painlessly moved normally. ROM can be active or passive, where the former is the full ROM when an individual moves the joint by themselves, and the latter is full ROM when the joint is moved by an external force, such as another person or the same individual using any assistive devices. When ROM at a particular joint is limited compared to normal ROM, joints can be classified as hypomobile, and when ROM is greater than normal ROM, joints can be classified as hypermobile.

The next step following understanding movement terminology is to comprehend the range in which these joints move. Predominant synovial joints move in angular fashion, and their range of motion (ROM) can be measured using a device called a goniometer and quantified in degrees. The goniometer is used by clinicians and health care professionals to assess and identify normal ROM as well any limited ROM due to musculoskeletal or neurological pathologies. Assessing ROM at all or specific joints of interest can aid not only in diagnosis but also in rehabilitation and prognosis of the pathological condition.

All individuals vary in size, shape, and form. Such variations are evident between sex, age, race, geographical locations, and genetic predispositions. Anthropometric measurements among the entire population follow a typical normal distribution bell curve, based on normative data. Assessing anthropometry right—from newborns to healthy adults to elderly individuals—allows us to make predictions and draw specific conclusions in various aspects of health, such as musculoskeletal or neurological pathologies, nutrition and malnutrition, and functional health status, based on an individual's body shape, size, and form.

REAL-WORLD APPLICATIONS

Assessment and measurement of both goniometric joint ROM and body anthropometry are widely used in settings such as clinics, rehabilitation, athletic training, fitness centers, sports performance centers, and occupational wellness centers. ROM measurements can aid in diagnosing a clinical condition such as a limited ROM due to a rotator cuff pathology in an elderly individual caused by aging and wear and tear, hyperextension of the knee joint after an athlete's anterior cruciate ligament injury caused by contact or plant and cut mechanisms, or hypoextension of an employee's wrist joint due to a carpal tunnel syndrome caused by repeated movements due to the nature of the occupation. Anthropometric measures allow us to predict the impact of the individual's body size, shape, and form on injury risk and degree of performance.

Goniometry Measurements

Equipment

- Paper
- Pencil or pen
- 360° goniometer
- Tape measure
- Calculator
- Individual laboratory report

Upper and Lower Extremity ROM Measurements

An important aspect of assessing ROM in clinical conditions is to know what normal ROM in all joints is. This lab activity will focus on measuring normal ROM available for each movement of each joint of interest in the upper and lower extremities.

For this lab, you will be making a series of goniometric measures on a participant for the major synovial joints in the both the upper and lower extremities and answering several questions related to your measurements.

The position of the participant for measuring ROM for each joint and each degree of freedom of movement, as well as the corresponding goniometer position are listed for the major joints of upper and lower extremity. Please follow the procedures and guidelines and measure the normal available ROM for the joints and movements listed. If there is any previous participant history of musculoskeletal injuries, please make a note of the injury, side, joint affected, and time line of the injury.

Using a participant, complete the normal ROM measurements for the joints listed in tables 2.1 and 2.2 on the individual laboratory report. Ensure participant and goniometer position for corresponding ROM measurements are as indicated in the tables.

Step 1: Position the participant corresponding to the joint intended for ROM measurement, along with the joint of interest in anatomical neutral position.

Step 2: Place the axis of the goniometer on the joint axis or corresponding bony landmark identified, align the stationary arm with a body segment that is not moving, and align the movable arm with the bone and body segment that moves. For each joint measurement, instruct the participant to move through the full ROM and move the moveable arm of the goniometer to align parallel with the body segment that moves.

Step 3: Measure the angle indicated in the goniometer and record the measurements in tables 2.1 and 2.2 on the individual laboratory report.

> This lab activity is accompanied by video demonstrations of goniometer measurements on HK*Propel*.

Question Set 2.1

1. Complete the normal ROM for each movement for each joint in both an upper and a lower extremity.

2. How does the ROM at each joint compare with normative data available through associations such as the American Medical Association and the American Academy of Orthopaedic Surgeons?

3. Did any particular joint have hypermobility or hypomobility?

4. What was the type of end feel present for each of the joint movements?

LABORATORY ACTIVITY 2.1

INDIVIDUAL LABORATORY REPORT

Name or ID number: _____ Date: _____

Tester: _____ Time: _____

Table 2.1 Upper Extremity

| Joint | Movement performed and measured | Participant position | GONIOMETER POSITION | | | Normal ROM | |
			Axis	Stationary arm	Movable arm		
Shoulder	Flexion	Supine lying	Lateral aspect of acromion process	Parallel to the midaxillary line	Aligned parallel with the humerus	0-180	
	Extension	Prone lying	Lateral aspect of acromion process	Parallel to the midaxillary line	Aligned parallel with the humerus	0-60 from neutral	
	Abduction	Supine lying	Anterior aspect of acromion process	Parallel to the sternum	Aligned parallel with the humerus	0-180	
	Adduction	Supine lying	Anterior aspect of acromion process	Parallel to the sternum	Aligned parallel with the humerus	0-45 from neutral	
	Internal rotation	Supine lying, shoulder at 90° abduction and elbow at 90° flexion	Olecranon process of ulna	Perpendicular to the floor	Aligned with ulna	0-70	
	External rotation	Supine lying, shoulder at 90° abduction and elbow at 90° flexion	Olecranon process of ulna	Perpendicular to the floor	Aligned with ulna	0-90	
Elbow	Flexion	Supine lying, shoulder anatomic neutral	Lateral epicondyle of the humerus	Parallel to the humerus	Aligned with the radius	0-150	
	Extension	Supine lying, shoulder anatomic neutral	Lateral epicondyle of the humerus	Parallel to the humerus	Aligned with the radius	150-0	
Wrist	Flexion	Sitting with forearm on table and hand hanging at the end of the table	Lateral part of the wrist joint	Parallel to the ulna	Aligned with the 5th metacarpal	0-80	
	Extension	Sitting with forearm on table and hand hanging at the end of the table	Lateral part of the wrist joint	Parallel to the ulna	Aligned with the 5th metacarpal	0-70	

(continued)

From J. Garner, C. Allen, H. Chander, and A. Knight, *Applied Biomechanics Laboratory Manual*. (Champaign, IL: Human Kinetics, 2023).

Table 2.1 *(continued)*

| Joint | Movement performed and measured | Participant position | GONIOMETER POSITION | | | Normal ROM | |
			Axis	Stationary arm	Movable arm		
	Radial deviation	Sitting with forearm on table and hand hanging at the end of the table	Capitate	Parallel to the forearm	Aligned with the 3rd metacarpal	0-20	
	Ulnar deviation	Sitting with forearm on table and hand hanging at the end of the table	Capitate	Parallel to the forearm	Aligned with the 3rd metacarpal	0-30	

Table 2.2 Lower Extremity

| Joint | Movement performed and measured | Participant position | GONIOMETER POSITION | | | Normal ROM (degrees) | |
			Axis	Stationary arm	Movable arm		
Hip	Flexion	Supine lying with knee flexion allowed during testing	Lateral aspect of the greater trochanter	Parallel to the midline of the pelvis	Aligned with the femur	0-120	
	Extension	Prone lying with knee flexion allowed during testing	Lateral aspect of the greater trochanter	Parallel to the midline of the pelvis	Aligned with the femur	0-30	
	Abduction	Supine lying with knee in extension	Anterior aspect of the anterior superior iliac spine	Parallel to the midline of the pelvis	Aligned with femur	0-45	
	Adduction	Supine lying with knee in extension	Anterior aspect of the anterior superior iliac spine	Parallel to the midline of the pelvis	Aligned with the femur	0-30 from neutral	
	Internal rotation	High sitting on table, with hip and knee at 90° flexion	Center of the patella	Perpendicular to the floor	Aligned with the tibia	0-45	
	External rotation	High sitting on table, with hip and knee at 90° flexion	Center of the patella	Perpendicular to the floor	Aligned with the tibia	0-45	
Knee	Flexion	Prone lying position	Lateral epicondyle of the femur	Parallel to the femur	Aligned with the fibula	0-150	
	Extension	Prone lying position	Lateral epicondyle of the femur	Parallel to the femur	Aligned with the fibula	150-0	

From J. Garner, C. Allen, H. Chander, and A. Knight, *Applied Biomechanics Laboratory Manual.* (Champaign, IL: Human Kinetics, 2023).

| Joint | Movement performed and measured | Participant position | GONIOMETER POSITION | | | Normal ROM (degrees) | |
			Axis	Stationary arm	Movable arm		
Ankle	Dorsiflexion	High sitting on table, with hip and knee at 90° flexion, ankle at anatomic neutral	Lateral malleolus of the fibula	Parallel to the fibula	Aligned with the 5th metatarsal	0-20	
	Plantar flexion	High sitting on table, with hip and knee at 90° flexion, ankle at anatomic neutral	Lateral malleolus of the fibula	Parallel to the fibula	Aligned with the 5th metatarsal	0-50	
	Inversion	High sitting on table, with hip and knee at 90° flexion, ankle at anatomic neutral. Can be done in prone lying position.	Anterior aspect of feet in between the medial and lateral malleoli	Parallel to the tibia	Aligned with the 3rd metatarsal	0-35	
	Eversion	High sitting on table, with hip and knee at 90° flexion, ankle at anatomic neutral. Can be done in prone lying position.	Anterior aspect of feet in between the medial and lateral malleoli	Parallel to the tibia	Aligned with the 3rd metatarsal	0-15	

From J. Garner, C. Allen, H. Chander, and A. Knight, *Applied Biomechanics Laboratory Manual*. (Champaign, IL: Human Kinetics, 2023).

Anthropometry Measurements

Equipment

- Paper
- Pencil or pen
- Tape measure
- Calculator
- Individual laboratory report
- Group laboratory report

Anthropometry

Anthropometry refers to the study of human body measurement and plays an important role in biomechanics, as well as industrial design, clothing design, ergonomics, and architecture.

For this laboratory activity, you will be making a series of anthropometric measures on yourself and a participant. You will also be making a series of calculations based on these measures and answering several questions related to your measures and calculations.

This lab activity is split into three steps that include measurements of basic overall body anthropometry followed by calculations in each of the sections.

Step 1: Fill out section I of the individual laboratory report and complete the calculations.

Step 2: Work with a partner and use the tools provided to make most of the anthropometric measures indicated in the diagram that follows. Record your measurements and complete the calculations in section II of the individual laboratory report (figure 2.1).

Step 3: Combine the data from the entire class to calculate averages for the same measures on the group laboratory report. Only the fraction of standing height is necessary.

> This lab activity is accompanied by video demonstrations of anthropometric measurements on HK*Propel.*
>
> WWW

Question Set 2.2

1. The Centers for Disease Control and Prevention states that body mass index (BMI) provides a reliable indicator for body fatness for most people and is used to screen for weight categories that may lead to health problems. It is also reported in some research studies as a tool for describing the characteristics of the sample being tested. A person whose BMI is below 18.5 is considered underweight. A BMI between 18.5 and 24.9 is normal. A BMI between 25.0 and 29.9 is overweight, and 30.0 and above is obese. In general, is BMI a valid biomechanical measure for college students? Explain your answer.

2. How well does your data match up with the diagram?

3. How well does the group data match up with the diagram?

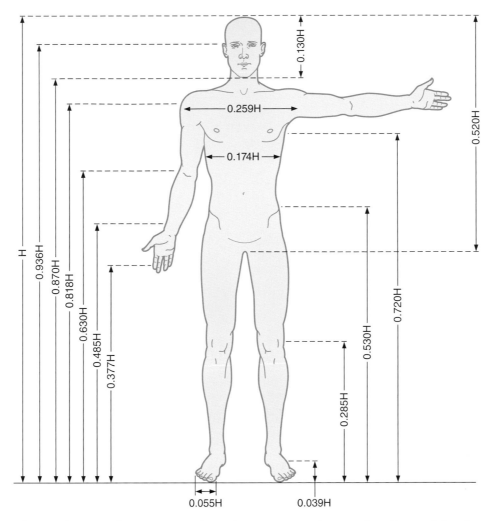

Figure 2.1 Body segment lengths expressed as a fraction of body height H.

Adapted from Drillis and Contini (1966).

4. The anthropometric data commonly used to create biomechanical models in modern laboratories typically come from studies performed in the 1800s and 1900s. In general, how have humans in the United States changed over the past 100 to 150 years? Why would any change have occurred?

5. Is it acceptable for biomechanics researchers to use these old anthropometric measures? Explain your answer, including a discussion of the limitations of the data discussed in class along with your comparisons of your individual and group data to the previously published values.

LABORATORY ACTIVITY 2.2

INDIVIDUAL LABORATORY REPORT

Name or ID number: _____ Date: _____

Tester: _____ Time: _____

Section I

What is your height? _____ in. _____ m (1 in. = 2.54 cm)

What is your weight? _____ lb _____ N (1 lb = 4.45 N)

What is your mass? _____ kg (1 kg = 2.2 lb, gravity = 9.81 m/s^2)

What is your BMI? _____ kg/m^2

BMI = (mass in kg)/(height in m × height in m) (1 kg = 2.2 lb, gravity = 9.81 m/s^2)

Section II

Head height: _____ in. _____ fraction of standing height

Spine to shoulder: _____ in. _____ fraction of standing height

Shoulder to elbow: _____ in. _____ fraction of standing height

Elbow to wrist: _____ in. _____ fraction of standing height

Hand length: _____ in. _____ fraction of standing height

Shoulder to shoulder: _____ in. _____ fraction of standing height

Rib cage width: _____ in. _____ fraction of standing height

Hip width: _____ in. _____ fraction of standing height

Foot breadth: _____ in. _____ fraction of standing height

Foot length: _____ in. _____ fraction of standing height

Floor to ankle: _____ in. _____ fraction of standing height

Floor to knee: _____ in. _____ fraction of standing height

Floor to hip: _____ in. _____ fraction of standing height

Floor to fingertip: _____ in. _____ fraction of standing height

Floor to wrist: _____ in. _____ fraction of standing height

Floor to elbow: _____ in. _____ fraction of standing height

Floor to shoulder: _____ in. _____ fraction of standing height

Floor to chin: _____ in. _____ fraction of standing height

Floor to eye level: _____ in. _____ fraction of standing height

From J. Garner, C. Allen, H. Chander, and A. Knight, *Applied Biomechanics Laboratory Manual*. (Champaign, IL: Human Kinetics, 2023).

LABORATORY ACTIVITY 2.2

GROUP LABORATORY REPORT

Name or ID number: _____ Date: _____

Tester: _____ Time: _____

Group data

Head height: _____ fraction of standing height

Spine to shoulder: _____ fraction of standing height

Shoulder to elbow: _____ fraction of standing height

Elbow to wrist: _____ fraction of standing height

Hand length: _____ fraction of standing height

Shoulder to shoulder: _____ fraction of standing height

Rib cage width: _____ fraction of standing height

Hip width: _____ fraction of standing height

Foot breadth: _____ fraction of standing height

Foot length: _____ fraction of standing height

Floor to ankle: _____ fraction of standing height

Floor to knee: _____ fraction of standing height

Floor to hip: _____ fraction of standing height

Floor to fingertip: _____ fraction of standing height

Floor to wrist: _____ fraction of standing height

Floor to elbow: _____ fraction of standing height

Floor to shoulder: _____ fraction of standing height

Floor to chin: _____ fraction of standing height

Floor to eye level: _____ fraction of standing height

From J. Garner, C. Allen, H. Chander, and A. Knight, *Applied Biomechanics Laboratory Manual.* (Champaign, IL: Human Kinetics, 2023).

Center of Mass Location

Equipment

- Paper
- Pencil or pen
- Tape measure
- Calculator
- Completed individual and group laboratory reports from laboratory activity 2.2
- Individual laboratory report for laboratory activity 2.3

Center of Mass

In addition to the measurements in laboratory activity 2.2, we can also use this data to calculate the center of mass location for different body segments. This is useful for determining the moment of inertia of a segment or limb or for performing an inverse dynamics analysis. While that may be beyond the scope of an undergraduate biomechanics lab, it is still beneficial to know how to calculate the center of mass for different body segments. Several different researchers have estimated the location of the center of mass for our different limb segments (Zatsiorsky et al., 1990; de Leva, 1996), and we can use these percentages to approximate the center of mass location based on the previous measurements you have taken.

Step 1: Convert the segment lengths you have previously calculated into centimeters.

Step 2: Multiply this length in centimeters by the center of mass location that is given for each segment. One inch is equal to 2.54 cm. The estimates are different for males and females, so make sure to use the correct center of mass percentage.

Step 3: Using a tape measure, measure the length of the thigh and shank in centimeters.

Step 4: Multiply the thigh and shank measurements by the center of mass location percentage for each segment, making sure to use the correct percentage for the person's sex. Since these are listed as percentages, you will need to multiply each percentage by 0.01 before you multiply the percentage by the segment length. For example, we will determine the center of mass location for a male forearm using table 2.3. We will assume the length of the male's forearm is 10.67 in., which is 27.1 cm (10.67 in. × 2.54 cm/in.). The location of the center of mass for a male forearm is 45.74% of the length of the forearm, from the proximal end of the segment. Therefore, we would multiply the length of the forearm, which is 27.1 cm, by 0.4574 (remember to multiply the center of mass location percentage by 0.01), which would reveal the location of the center of mass for this male forearm is 12.40 cm from the proximal end of the segment.

Table 2.3 Center of Mass Locations for Selected Segments for Males and Females

Segment	Center of mass location for males (%)	Center of mass location for females (%)
Upper arm	57.72	57.54
Forearm	45.74	45.59
Hand	79.00	74.74
Thigh	40.95	36.12
Shank	44.59	44.16
Foot	44.15	40.14

LABORATORY ACTIVITY 2.3

INDIVIDUAL LABORATORY REPORT

Name or ID number: _____ Date: _____

Tester: _____ Time: _____

Upper arm (shoulder to elbow length): _____ in. = _____ cm × _____ center of mass percentage = _____ cm (center of mass location from the proximal end of the segment)

Forearm (elbow to wrist length): _____ in. = _____ cm × _____ center of mass percentage = _____ cm (center of mass location from the proximal end of the segment)

Hand length: _____ in. = _____ cm × _____ center of mass percentage = _____ cm (center of mass location from the proximal end of the segment)

Thigh length: _____ in. = _____ cm × _____ center of mass percentage = _____ cm (center of mass location from the proximal end of the segment)

Shank length: _____ in. = _____ cm × _____ center of mass percentage = _____ cm (center of mass location from the proximal end of the segment)

Foot length: _____ in. = _____ cm × _____ center of mass percentage = _____ cm (center of mass location from the proximal end of the segment)

From J. Garner, C. Allen, H. Chander, and A. Knight, *Applied Biomechanics Laboratory Manual.* (Champaign, IL: Human Kinetics, 2023).

Linear Kinematics in One Direction

Objectives

- Understand the principles of linear kinematics in one direction.
- Investigate the mechanical components of linear kinematics in one direction.
- Apply the basic principles of linear kinematics in one direction across disciplines.

DEFINITIONS

position (p)—An object's location in space. Knowing this position, whether in a closed lab motion-capture environment or in the middle of a soccer pitch, is vitally important to all linear kinematic calculations. Mechanically, this serves as our reference location in order to calculate the derivatives of linear motion.

displacement (s, Δp)—The straight-line difference in positions between two time points. In most settings, this will be in a specific direction and be defined by the starting point (reference position) and the final position. Displacement is a vector quantity and may be negative if the direction of motion requires movement in the negative direction.

velocity (v)—The rate of change in the position of an object, with respect to time in a specific direction. In practical terms, velocity tells us how fast or slow a person or object is moving and the direction in which the person or object is moving.

acceleration (a)—The rate of change of the linear velocity. This can also be defined as the rate at which an object is speeding up or slowing down in a straight line.

CALCULATING LINEAR KINEMATICS

Calculating Displacement

Displacement is calculated by determining the difference between the object's final and initial position:

$$\Delta p = p_2 - p_1$$

Linear displacement may be measured in any linear unit (e.g., meters, feet, yards, miles). It may be expressed as Δp or s.

Calculating Velocity

In order to calculate velocity, the researcher must have several pieces of information to accurately measure or calculate velocity. These include:

- **final position**—The final point of the movement of interest, often referred to as p_f.
- **initial position**—The beginning point of the movement of interest, often referred to as p_i.
- **time**—The time taken for the motion of interest to occur, referred as δt or t.

Velocity is calculated by dividing the change in position, or displacement, by the time change:

$$v = \frac{\Delta p}{\Delta t}$$

Linear velocity may be measured in any linear unit per unit time (e.g., meters per second, miles per hour). As it is considered the first-time derivative of displacement, it is also a vector quantity. In this case the positive or negative sign indicates the direction of movement, not the magnitude.

Calculating Linear Acceleration

Linear acceleration is calculated by dividing the difference between the object's final velocity and its initial velocity by the time it took to move between those velocities. More simply, it is the change in linear velocity divided by time. In order to calculate velocity, the researcher must have several pieces of information to accurately measure or calculate velocity. These include:

- **final linear velocity**—This is the velocity at the final point of the movement of interest and is often referred to as v_f.
- **initial linear velocity**—This is the velocity at the beginning point of the movement of interest and is often referred to as v_i.
- **time**—This is the time taken for the motion of interest to occur and is referred as Δt or t.

$$a = \frac{\Delta v}{\Delta t} = \frac{v_f - v_i}{\Delta t}$$

The most common units of measure for linear acceleration include meters per second per second (m/s/s or m/s²), feet per second per second (ft/s/s or ft/s²), or any other velocity per unit time.

LABORATORY INTRODUCTION

Linear motion is often referred to as translation and occurs when a point (or all points) move in a straight line in the same direction. In human movement, we may have both linear and angular motion but must be able to differentiate between the two in order to properly analyze the motions. Although a 100 m sprinter must be able to rotate their joints to produce movement, the winner of the race is determined by who can move their body to the finish line the fastest. It is understood that a lot of angular movements cause the motion of the entire body, and we care only about how the body, as a whole, moves from the starting line to the finish line in one direction, hopefully in a straight line. It is this linear movement that we will focus on in laboratory activity 3.1.

In running events, a competitive athlete's goal is to cover a given distance in the shortest possible time. From a biomechanics perspective, the goal is to cover the distance with the highest possible average velocity or speed. This is a simple example of how our fundamental principles of linear kinematics become useful in our understanding of performance. By describing various kinematic aspects of running, we can gain some information about strengths and weaknesses in an athlete's performance that may lead to better running times or a reduced potential for injury. Laboratory activity 3.1 focuses on some of the most basic descriptors of running performance: time, displacement, velocity, and acceleration. This activity deals with sprinting kinematics, although the basic principles would apply to any form of running.

This purpose of this activity is to investigate patterns of linear displacement, velocity, and acceleration for two 25 m sprints in opposite directions.

To determine displacement in meters, we will break the 25 m sprints up into 2.5 m intervals (0-2.5 m, 5-7.5 m, . . ., 22.5-25 m). You will need to consider both the displacement for each interval (which will always be 2.5 m) and the accumulated displacement, which will start at 0 m and increase to 25 m or decrease to −25 m at the end of the sprint. Note: These values can be negative depending on the direction of the run.

The highest average velocity over the whole run determines who wins the race. However, average velocity over the whole run provides a general snapshot of the movement but does not give specific details from the standpoint of examining the runner's performance and racing strategy. We will approximate the runner's instantaneous velocity by calculating the average velocity over each 2.5 m interval, and then plot the results to see how velocity changes over the 25 m. Note: These values can be negative.

The average acceleration over the whole run is even less informative than the average velocity. Again, we will approximate the runner's instantaneous acceleration by calculating the average acceleration over every 2.5 m interval and plot the results. Note: These values can be negative.

Linear Kinematics of a Running Event

Equipment

- Paper
- Pencil or pen
- Calculator
- Stopwatch
- Tape measure
- Cones
- Whistle
- Individual laboratory report
- Group laboratory report

Displacement, Velocity, and Acceleration Profiles for Sprinting

Step 1: Set up a 25 m run course (in a lab or where space allows) with cones or other type of marker placed every 2.5 m (see figure 3.1). Students will work together to collect descriptive data for four student volunteers (runners 1 to 4) who will sprint the course at full effort. (Be sure that the runners stretch, warm up, and wear proper running footwear and athletic clothing.)

Step 2: Set up one student as the starter positioned at the starting line.

Step 3: Position at least one person at each of the cones to record the times as the runner passes by.

Step 4: The starter will make sure both the runner and the timers are ready for each trial.

Step 5: Runner 1 will begin at the 0 m mark for the first trial from a standing or crouched position. For each trial, a starter will give a loud ready-set-go sequence of verbal commands, or blow a whistle, at which time the runner will initiate his or her sprint to the finish line, and all timers will begin timing the performance.

Step 6: As runner 1 passes each 2.5 m position, the timers at those locations will stop their watches and record the number in the appropriate cell on the group laboratory report.

Step 7: For the second run, runner 2 will start at the 25 m mark and run to the 0 m mark, thereby running in the negative direction.

Step 8: This same sequence will then be repeated for runners 3 and 4, and the data will be recorded in the appropriate cell on the group laboratory report.

This lab activity is accompanied by a video demonstration on HK*Propel*.

www

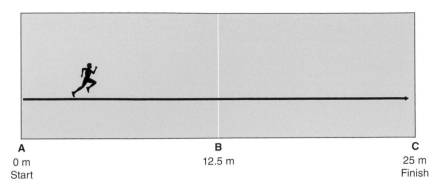

A
0 m
Start

B
12.5 m

C
25 m
Finish

Figure 3.1 Example of a 25 m run course.

Laboratory Report

Use the average temporal data from the group laboratory report to complete the information on the individual laboratory report in tables 3.1 to 3.4 before the next laboratory. These tables can either be filled out at the end of this document or typed up in Word or Excel. In addition to finishing these tables, you will answer the following questions.

Question Set 3.1

1. During each run, identify at which interval the following occurred (two answers each):

   a. Peak velocity (positive or negative, depending on direction of running)

   b. Peak acceleration

   c. Peak negative acceleration

2. In order to increase your running velocity, you will need to cover a greater displacement in a given time or achieve the same displacement in a lesser amount of time. One way of doing this is to increase your stride length, but at some point, you will not be able to lengthen your stride anymore as your legs are not long enough. What other kinematic variable discussed in class will increase your running velocity?

3. If we recreated the 25 m run for this lab but placed a wall at the end of the 25 m, how would this change our results? What do you think would change about our data?

GROUP LABORATORY REPORT

Data From Runners

Runner 1   Temporal Data

Position (m)	Time (s)
0	0
2.5	
5	
7.5	
10	
12.5	
15	
17.5	
20	
22.5	
25	

Runner 1   Temporal Data

Position (m)	Time (s)
0	0
2.5	
5	
7.5	
10	
12.5	
15	
17.5	
20	
22.5	
25	

Runner 2   Temporal Data

Position (m)	Time (s)
25	0
22.5	
20	
17.5	
15	
12.5	
10	
7.5	
5	
2.5	
0	

Runner 2   Temporal Data

Position (m)	Time (s)
25	0
22.5	
20	
17.5	
15	
12.5	
10	
7.5	
5	
2.5	
0	

From J. Garner, C. Allen, H. Chander, and A. Knight, *Applied Biomechanics Laboratory Manual.* (Champaign, IL: Human Kinetics, 2023).

LABORATORY ACTIVITY 3.1

INDIVIDUAL LABORATORY REPORT

Name or ID number: _____ Date: _____

Tester: _____ Time: _____

To calculate the velocities and accelerations, you must use the equations listed in the Calculating Linear Kinematics section.

Laboratory Activity 3.1 Table 1   Runner 1 Linear Kinematics

Time (s)	Cumulative displacement (m)	Change in time (s)	Interval displacement (m)	Velocity (m/s)	Change in velocity (m/s)	Acceleration (m/s^2)
0	0	0	0	0	0	0
	2.5					
	5					
	7.5					
	10					
	12.5					
	15					
	17.5					
	20					
	22.5					
	25					

Laboratory Activity 3.1 Table 2   Runner 2 Linear Kinematics

Time (s)	Cumulative displacement (m)	Change in time (s)	Interval displacement (m)	Velocity (m/s)	Change in velocity (m/s)	Acceleration (m/s^2)
0	25	0	0	0	0	0
	22.5					
	20					
	17.5					
	15					
	12.5					
	10					
	7.5					
	5					
	2.5					
	0					

From J. Garner, C. Allen, H. Chander, and A. Knight, *Applied Biomechanics Laboratory Manual*. (Champaign, IL: Human Kinetics, 2023).

Laboratory Activity 3.1 Table 3 Runner 3 Linear Kinematics

Time (s)	Cumulative displacement (m)	Change in time (s)	Interval displacement (m)	Velocity (m/s)	Change in velocity (m/s)	Acceleration (m/s^2)
0	0	0	0	0	0	0
	2.5					
	5					
	7.5					
	10					
	12.5					
	15					
	17.5					
	20					
	22.5					
	25					

Laboratory Activity 3.1 Table 4 Runner 4 Linear Kinematics

Time (s)	Cumulative displacement (m)	Change in time (s)	Interval displacement (m)	Velocity (m/s)	Change in velocity (m/s)	Acceleration (m/s^2)
0	25	0	0	0	0	0
	22.5					
	20					
	17.5					
	15					
	12.5					
	10					
	7.5					
	5					
	2.5					
	0					

From J. Garner, C. Allen, H. Chander, and A. Knight, *Applied Biomechanics Laboratory Manual*. (Champaign, IL: Human Kinetics, 2023).

Linear Kinematics in Two Directions

Objectives

- Understand the principles of linear kinematics in two directions.
- Understand the mechanical components of linear kinematics in two directions.
- Apply the basic principles of linear kinematics in two directions across disciplines.

DEFINITIONS

distance (d)—The amount of ground covered: $\Delta d = d_2 - d_1$

Displacement (s or Δp)—Change in position: $\Delta p = p_2 - p_1$

speed (m/s)—The rate in change in distance, with respect to time: $s = \dfrac{\Delta d}{\Delta t}$

velocity (m/s)—The rate of change in position, with respect to time: $v = \dfrac{\Delta p}{\Delta t}$

acceleration (m/s²)—The rate of change of velocity, with respect to time: $a = \dfrac{\Delta v}{\Delta t}$

In this laboratory, we will investigate patterns of distance, linear displacement, velocity, and acceleration for two 10 m shuttle runs.

We will have the runners complete a 10 m shuttle, which will be broken down into intervals of 5 m. You will need to consider the **distance** for each interval (which will always be 5 m) and the total distance, which will be 20 m. These values will be positive because of the scalar property of distance.

We will break the 10 m shuttle up into 5 m intervals (0-5 m, 5-10 m, 10-5 m, 5-0 m). You will need to consider both the **displacement** for each interval (which will always be 5 m either positive or negative) and the accumulated displacement, which will start at 0 m, increase to 10 m, and return to 0 m at the end of the shuttle. These values will be both positive and negative because of the change in direction.

For sprinting, the highest average **speed** over the whole run determines who wins the race. However, average speed over the whole run is not that informative from the standpoint of examining the runner's performance, racing strategy, and direction. In this laboratory, we will approximate the runner's instantaneous speed by calculating the average speed over each 5 m interval and see how speed changes over the course of the shuttle. These values will be positive because of the scalar property of speed.

For sprinting, the highest average **velocity** over the whole run determines who wins the race. However, average velocity over the whole run is not that informative from the standpoint of examining the runner's performance and racing strategy. In this lab, we will approximate the runner's instantaneous velocity by calculating the average velocity over each 5 m interval and see how velocity changes over the course of the shuttle. These values will be both positive and negative because of the change in direction.

The average **acceleration** over the whole run is even less informative than the average velocity. Again, we will approximate the runner's instantaneous acceleration by calculating the average acceleration over every 5 m interval. These values can be negative.

In a shuttle run, an athlete is asked to run from point A to point B, slow down, stop, turn round at point B, and then run back to point A. The distance covered during a shuttle run can vary, and the number of times the athlete has to change directions can vary as well. Unlike a sprint from point A to point B, which only requires an athlete to run in one direction, a shuttle run measures an athlete's ability to change directions.

A competitive athlete's goal is to complete the course or shuttle in the shortest possible time. From a biomechanics perspective, the goal is to complete the shuttle with the highest average speed over the entire shuttle run and to have the highest average velocity as the athlete moves from one point to the next. This laboratory focuses on building off the knowledge gained from previous labs and calculating some of the most basic descriptors of running performance—time, distance, speed, displacement, velocity, and acceleration. The lab deals with sprinting kinematics and changing of directions, although the basic principles would apply to any form of running.

RELATIONSHIP BETWEEN THE DIRECTION OF THE VELOCITY AND ACCELERATION VECTORS

During the first part of the shuttle run, from point A to point C, the person is running in the positive horizontal direction. Therefore, the person's displacement and velocity vectors will be in the positive direction. During the second part of the shuttle run, from point C to point E, the person is running in the negative direction, and their displacement and velocity vectors will

be in the negative direction.

To determine the direction of the acceleration vector, we have to examine if the person's velocity is increasing (speeding up) or decreasing (slowing down). First, we will examine the person's velocity as they move from point A to point C. At both of these points, the person's velocity will be 0 m/s. As the person moves from point A to point B, their velocity will increase from 0 m/s in the positive direction. This means that they are speeding up, and their velocity and acceleration vectors will both be positive. From point B to point C, the person will have to decrease their velocity as they near point C in order to slow down, stop, and turn the other direction. Although the person is slowing down, their velocity vector will still be positive (because they are still moving in the positive direction), but their acceleration vector will be negative. Next, let's examine the person's velocity as they move from point C to point A. At both of these points, their velocity will be 0 m/s. As the person moves from point C to point D, their velocity will increase from 0 m/s in the negative direction. Although the person is speeding up, in the negative direction, their velocity and acceleration vectors will both be negative. From point D to point E, the person will have to decrease their velocity as they near point E in order to slow down and stop. Although this person is slowing down and their velocity vector will still be negative, their acceleration vector will be positive.

We can conclude some important points from this. If a person is increasing velocity (speeding up), then their velocity and acceleration vectors will be in the same direction. If the person is moving in the positive direction, then both velocity and acceleration will be positive, and if the person is moving in the negative direction, then both the velocity and acceleration vectors will be negative. If a person is decreasing velocity (slowing down), then their velocity and acceleration vectors will be in the opposite direction. If the person is moving in the positive direction, then the velocity vector will be positive and the acceleration vector will be negative. If the person is moving in the negative direction, then the velocity vector will be negative and the acceleration vector will be positive.

Linear Kinematics of a Running Event in Two Directions

Equipment

- Paper
- Pencil or pen
- Calculator
- Stopwatches or stopwatch app
- Tape measure
- Tape
- Cones
- Whistle
- Group laboratory report
- Individual laboratory report (to be completed before next lab)

Displacement, Velocity, and Acceleration Profiles for Sprinting

Step 1: Set up a 10 m shuttle run course with tape placed every 5 m (see figure 4.1). Students will work together to collect data for four student volunteers (runners 1 to 4) who will sprint the course at full effort (be sure that the runners stretch, warm up, and wear proper running footwear and athletic clothing).

Step 2: Set up one student as the starter positioned at the starting line (A and E).

Step 3: Position two people at the at the 5 m mark (B and D) and one person at the 10 m mark (C) to record the times using stopwatches or a stopwatch app on a smartphone as the runner passes by.

Step 4: The starter will make sure runner 1 and the timers are ready.

Step 5: Runner 1 will begin at the 0 m mark for the first trial from a standing or crouched position. For each trial, a starter will give a loud ready-set-go sequence of verbal commands, at which time the runner will initiate his or her shuttle run to the finish line, and all timers will begin timing the performance.

Step 6: As the runner passes each 5 m position, a timer at that location will stop their watch and record the number in the appropriate cell in the group laboratory report. (Note: There are two people stationed at the 5 m position because the runner will pass this location twice, thus creating two different time points.)

Step 7: The same sequence will then be repeated for runners 2, 3, and 4, and the data will be recorded in the appropriate cells on the group laboratory report. The data from the first two runners will be used to complete

This lab activity is accompanied by a video demonstration on *HKPropel*.

WWW

the in-class portion of the individual laboratory report and the data from the last two runners will be used to complete the individual laboratory report before the next laboratory.

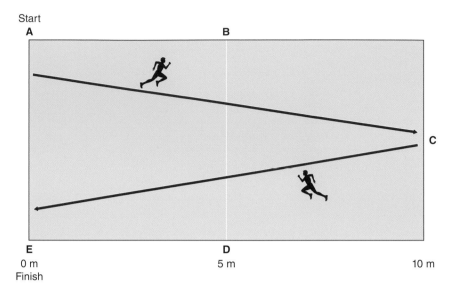

Start
A   B

E   D
0 m   5 m   10 m
Finish

Figure 4.1 Example of a 10 m shuttle run course.

Laboratory Report

Based on the average temporal data for runners 1 and 2, compute the following and record the fastest runners' results in laboratory activity 4.1 tables 1 and 2. To calculate the velocities and accelerations, you must use the equations listed in Definitions.

Using data for runners 3 and 4, you will complete laboratory activity 4.1 tables 3 and 4 for your next laboratory. Use the individual laboratory report to complete these tables. In addition to finishing these tables, you will answer the following questions.

Question Set 4.1

1. During each run, identify at which interval the following occurred (two answers each):

   a. Peak velocity (positive or negative, depending on direction of running)

   b. Peak acceleration

   c. Peak negative acceleration

2. We can calculate the average speed of the total shuttle by taking the total distance covered during the shuttle divided by the time it took to complete the shuttle. Calculate the average speed for both runners.

3. We can calculate the average velocity of the total shuttle by taking the final displacement during the shuttle divided by the time it took to complete the shuttle. Calculate the average velocity for both runners.

4. Are the numbers calculated for average speed (question 2) and average velocity (question 3) the same? If yes, why are they the same? If no, why are they different?

LABORATORY ACTIVITY 4.1

GROUP LABORATORY REPORT

Data From Runners

Runner 1 Shuttle Temporal Data

Position	Time (s)
A	0
B	
C	
D	
E	

Runner 3 Shuttle Temporal Data

Position	Time (s)
A	0
B	
C	
D	
E	

Runner 2 Shuttle Temporal Data

Position	Time (s)
A	0
B	
C	
D	
E	

Runner 4 Shuttle Temporal Data

Position	Time (s)
A	0
B	
C	
D	
E	

Laboratory Activity 4.1 Table 1 Runner 1 Shuttle Linear Kinematics

	Time (s)	Cumulative distance (m)	Cumulative displacement (m)	Change in time (s)	Interval distance (m)	Speed (m/s)	Interval displacement (m)	Velocity (m/s)	Change in velocity (m/s)	Acceleration (m/s²)
A	0	0	0	0	0	0	0	0	0	0
B		5	5							
C		10	10							
D		15	5							
E		20	0							

From J. Garner, C. Allen, H. Chander, and A. Knight, *Applied Biomechanics Laboratory Manual.* (Champaign, IL: Human Kinetics, 2023).

Laboratory Activity 4.1 Table 2   Runner 2 Shuttle Linear Kinematics

	Time (s)	Cumulative distance (m)	Cumulative displacement (m)	Change in time (s)	Interval distance (m)	Speed (m/s)	Interval displacement (m)	Velocity (m/s)	Change in velocity (m/s)	Acceleration (m/s²)
A	0	0	0	0	0	0	0	0	0	0
B		5	5							
C		10	10							
D		15	5							
E		20	0							

Laboratory Activity 4.1 Table 3   Runner 3 Shuttle Linear Kinematics

	Time (s)	Cumulative distance (m)	Cumulative displacement (m)	Change in time (s)	Interval distance (m)	Speed (m/s)	Interval displacement (m)	Velocity (m/s)	Change in velocity (m/s)	Acceleration (m/s²)
A	0	0	0	0	0	0	0	0	0	0
B		5	5							
C		10	10							
D		15	5							
E		20	0							

Laboratory Activity 4.1 Table 4   Runner 4 Shuttle Linear Kinematics

	Time (s)	Cumulative distance (m)	Cumulative displacement (m)	Change in time (s)	Interval distance (m)	Speed (m/s)	Interval displacement (m)	Velocity (m/s)	Change in velocity (m/s)	Acceleration (m/s²)
A	0	0	0	0	0	0	0	0	0	0
B		5	5							
C		10	10							
D		15	5							
E		20	0							

From J. Garner, C. Allen, H. Chander, and A. Knight, *Applied Biomechanics Laboratory Manual*. (Champaign, IL: Human Kinetics, 2023).

Projectile Motion: Jumping and Kicking

Objectives

- Understand the principles of projectile motion in regard to jumping and kicking and their application to human motion, particularly in the area of human performance.
- Describe the steps need to solve for the range and maximum height of the projectile.

DEFINITIONS

max height (in meters)—How high a person, ball, or other projectile travels from the ground to the apex; calculated using this formula: $\Delta^y p = {}^y v^2 / 2a$. To calculate the maximum height, you square the initial y velocity and then divide by 2 times acceleration due to gravity.

projectile—Any airborne body that is only subjected to gravity and wind resistance after it has left the ground.

range (in meters)—How far the projectile (such as a person or a ball) travels.

To calculate the range, you multiply the x velocity by the total time the projectile is in the air using this formula: $\Delta^x p = {}^x v t$.

trajectory—The path of a projectile; this will be in the shape of a parabola.

Often times in human movement, we become a projectile, such as when we jump, or we project an object, such as when we kick or throw a ball or hit a ball with a bat, racket, or club. Once an object is projected, it is only subjected to gravity, which causes a constant acceleration in the vertical direction of -9.81 m/s^2, and wind resistance. If we neglect wind resistance, which we will do initially, we can use the equations for constant acceleration provided here to calculate how far the projected person or object will travel (range) and what the person or object's maximum height will be.

- $\Delta p = v_i t + 1/2 a t^2$ (this can be used for either horizontal or vertical displacement)
- $v_f = v_i + at$; or $t = (v_f - v_i) / a$
- $v_f^2 = v_i^2 + 2a\Delta p$
- i = initial; f = final; Δp = displacement; v = velocity; a = acceleration; t = time

In order to use these equations, you must first break down the resultant velocity vector into its horizontal (x) and vertical (y) components. Then you can solve for the time the person or object will be in the air, how far the person or object will travel (range), and the person or object's maximum height (vertical displacement). There are some important things to remember when working projectile motion problems in which a person or object takes off and lands at the same height:

- Gravity acts in the negative vertical (y) direction. The acceleration due to gravity is -9.81 m/s^2. Gravity will reduce the vertical velocity of a person or object as it travels up toward the apex (the highest point of the trajectory) until it is 0 m/s at the apex. As the person or object travels toward the ground, gravity will increase its vertical velocity in the negative direction until it is equal to the person's vertical velocity at takeoff. For example, if a person's initial y velocity is 7 m/s, their y velocity at the apex will be 0 m/s, and the person's final y velocity right before landing will be −7 m/s.

- Since gravity only acts in the vertical direction, there is no acceleration of the person or object in the horizontal direction ($^{x}a = 0$ m/s²) if wind resistance is neglected. This means the horizontal, or x velocity of the person or object is constant throughout the entire trajectory. For example, if a person jumps with an initial x velocity of 4 m/s, his or her x velocity will be 4 m/s at any point along the trajectory.

- When solving for range, since the acceleration in the x direction is 0 m/s², you can use the equation $\Delta p = v_i t$ (range = x velocity multiplied by total time).

- The time it takes a person or object to travel from the ground to the apex is the same amount of time it takes the person or object to travel from the apex back to the ground (time up is equal to time down). For example, if it takes a person 0.5 seconds to travel from the ground to the apex of his or her jump, it will also take 0.5 s for the person to travel from the apex of his or her jump to the ground.

- When solving for time, only use the velocities in the vertical (y) direction and the acceleration in the vertical (y) direction. The acceleration in the vertical (y) direction will always be −9.81 m/s².

PROJECTILE MOTION PROCESS

When you are given the resultant velocity of a person or object and the angle at which the person or object leaves the ground, there is a four-step process to follow in order to solve for the range and the maximum height of the person or object. If you follow these steps and use the previous equations, it is a straightforward process. The following steps demonstrate how to work a projectile motion problem.:

1. Take the resultant velocity and angle and solve for the x and y components of the resultant velocity. This is where you will use the sine and cosine functions. For example, if you kicked a ball with a resultant velocity of 14 m/s at an angle 32° counterclockwise from the ground, you would use the following:

   a. x velocity: cos 32° (14 m/s) = 11.87 m/s

   b. y velocity: sin 32° (14 m/s) = 7.42 m/s

   In this example, x velocity is adjacent to the angle, and y velocity is opposite. That is why we are using the cosine function to solve for x velocity and the sine function to solve for the y velocity. Since we have an angle of 32°, the x velocity should be larger than the y velocity.

2. Solve for the time the ball is in the air. When solving for time, you only use the velocities and accelerations in the y (vertical) direction. We know that for a projectile motion problem the acceleration in the vertical direction will always be −9.81 m/s². We solved for the initial y velocity in step 1. As the person or object travels up towards the apex, its vertical velocity will decrease and at the apex the vertical velocity will be equal to 0 m/s. As the object comes down, its vertical velocity will increase in the negative direction until it is equal to its initial velocity. In our current problem, we know the initial y velocity is 7.42 m/s, the y velocity at the apex is 0 m/s, and the y velocity at the bottom is −7.42 m/s.

   To solve for time, we use the equation $t = (v_f - v_i) / a$. Again, when solving for time, we only use the velocities and acceleration in the vertical direction. We know that final y velocity is −7.42 m/s, initial y velocity is 7.41 m/s, and acceleration is −9.81 m/s². We just need to plug these numbers into our equation: $t = (-7.42$ m/s $- 7.42$ m/s$) / -9.81$ m/s². If we do the math, then time = 1.51 s. Since time up is equal to time down, we could divide this number by 2 to determine how long it took the person or object to go from the bottom to the apex and how long it took them to go from the apex to the bottom (time up = 0.755 s and time down = 0.755 s).

3. Now we can solve for range the range of the ball. The range is the horizontal (x) displacement. We can use the equation $\Delta p = v_i t + 1/2at^2$. Since the acceleration in the horizontal direction is 0 m/s² (remember, gravity only acts in the vertical direction), we can simplify this equation to read $\Delta p = v_i t$. Since this is horizontal displacement, we have to use our initial x velocity, which is 11.87 m/s. We just need to multiply this velocity by time to solve for the range:

$$\Delta^x p = (11.87 \text{ m/s})(1.51 \text{ s}) = 17.92 \text{ m}$$

This tells us the ball traveled 17.92 m from where it left the person's foot until it hit the ground again.

4. The last thing to solve for is the maximum height, or the height of the person or the ball from the ground at the apex. Since the ball is starting and landing at the same height, its vertical displacement over the entire trajectory is 0 m. We are only interested in the vertical displacement from the ground to the apex. The simplest way to work this step is to use this equation: $v_f^2 = v_i^2 + 2a\Delta p$. Since we are in the vertical direction again, we have to go back to our vertical velocities and vertical acceleration. We are only going from the ground to the apex, so the final vertical velocity will always be 0 m/s (at the apex). We calculated the initial vertical velocity in step 1; it was 7.42 m/s, and the acceleration in the vertical direction is −9.81 m/s² (due to gravity). Since our final velocity is 0 m/s (vertical velocity at the apex), we can rearrange this equation to read that max height is equal to the initial y velocity squared divided by 2 times the acceleration due to gravity. Looking at the equation that follows, h is our maximum height (vertical displacement from the ground to the apex), y_v is our initial y velocity, and a is the acceleration due to gravity.

5. $h = \dfrac{y_v^{\,2}}{2a_g}$

In our example, h = (7.42 m/s)² / (2*−9.81 m/s²), so h = 2.81 m. We can say that the ball that was kicked had a range of 17.92 m and a maximum height of 2.81 m.

APPLICATION OF PROJECTILE MOTION TO HUMAN MOVEMENT AND PERFORMANCE

The principles of projectile motion can be used to improve human performance, especially jumping, kicking, throwing, and striking objects. The trajectory of the person or object will be parabolic—the overall shape of the parabola will be dependent on the velocity of the person when he or she leaves the ground or the object when it is kicked, thrown, or struck. The magnitude and direction, specifically, the angle of takeoff, release, or contact, are the primary factors that influence the shape of the parabola. For a high jump, the athlete experiences a large amount of vertical displacement and a relatively small amount of horizontal displacement. This is accomplished by the athlete applying most of the force into the ground in the vertical direction, which produces a relatively large angle of takeoff (between 75 and 85 degrees). A basketball player can change the shape of the parabola by altering the release angle for his or her jump shot. The hammer throw is an event where the athlete seeks to maximize horizontal displacement of the hammer, so their release angle should be close to 45°. The same principle would apply to a broad jump or long jump (also sometimes called a horizontal jump), in which the jumper takes off and lands at the same height (figure 5.1). The athlete should attempt to leave the ground at a 45° angle in order to maximize horizontal displacement (range).

In this laboratory, we have neglected the influence of air resistance on the trajectory of a projectile. If this is factored in, it will reduce the horizontal velocity of the projectile and reduce the range of the projectile. The main resistance that fluid in the air provides to the horizontal velocity and range of a projectile is drag force. Drag force has a direction parallel to the direction

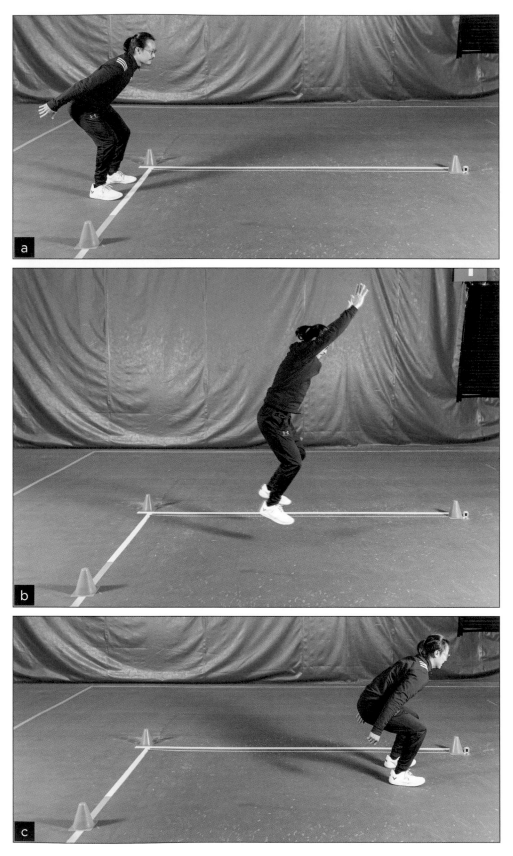

Figure 5.1 The (a) beginning, (b) apex, and (c) landing of a broad jump.

of fluid flow around the object. There is a direct method to determining the amount of drag force on an object, but you must calculate the projected area of the projectile and the velocity of the fluid relative to the object. A simpler method is to assume that air resistance will cause a linear reduction in the horizontal velocity of a projectile during its trajectory, in which case the final horizontal velocity will be equal to 0 m/s. Based on this assumption, you can take the initial horizontal velocity that was calculated and divide it by 2. For example, if a baseball is hit with an initial horizontal velocity of 35 m/s, and it is in the air for 7.5 seconds, without factoring in air resistance, the range of the baseball would be 262.5 m, which is approximately 861 feet. This is a much greater range than a home run in major league baseball. However, if you factor in air resistance by taking the initial horizontal velocity of 35 m/s and dividing it by 2, you then get a distance of 131.25 m, which is approximately 430 feet, and more representative of an actual home run.

Projectile Motion: Jumping

Equipment

- Video camera (a smartphone camera will work)
- Motion-analysis software such as Dartfish or MaxTRAQ
- Individual laboratory report

Calculating the Range and Maximum Height of a Broad Jump

Step 1: Place a strip of tape down on the floor where a volunteer will begin a broad jump.

Step 2: Position a second participant to video record the jump in the sagittal plane. They can use a video camera or the camera on their smartphone.

Step 3: The first participant should perform a broad jump, where they attempt to jump as far as possible.

Step 4: The second participant records the jump.

Step 5: Using a software program such as Dartfish or MaxTRAQ, you can calculate the angle of takeoff and the initial resultant velocity. You can then use those numbers to solve for the calculations in the individual laboratory report. If your lab is not equipped with this software, you can use the following hypothetical data to solve for the aforementioned variables:

A person jumps with a resultant velocity of 4.5 m/s at an angle 54° counterclockwise from the horizontal.

INDIVIDUAL LABORATORY REPORT

Name or ID number: _____ _____ Date: _____ _

Tester: _____ _____ Time: _____

Angle of takeoff: _____

Initial resultant velocity: _____

X component of velocity: _____

Y component of velocity: _____

Time the person is in the air: _____

Range of the person: _____

Maximum height of the person: _____

From J. Garner, C. Allen, H. Chander, and A. Knight, *Applied Biomechanics Laboratory Manual.* (Champaign, IL: Human Kinetics, 2023).

Projectile Motion: Kicking

Equipment

- Net
- Soccer ball
- Video camera or smartphone
- Motion-analysis software such as Dartfish or MaxTRAQ
- Individual laboratory report

Calculating the Range and Maximum Height of a Kicked Ball

Step 1: Choose two student volunteers to kick a soccer ball into the net in the classroom while it is being filmed from the sagittal plane. Lab instructors will be in charge of using the videos to obtain the resultant velocity and angle of the soccer ball kick. Place a strip of tape on the floor where they will begin the kicking motion.

Step 2: Choose one student volunteer to video the kick in the sagittal plane. They can use a video camera or the camera on their smartphone. The person will need to position the camera on the same side as the kicking leg.

Step 3: Instruct the kickers to kick the ball as far as they can.

Step 4: The second participant will record the kick.

Step 5: Using a software program such as Dartfish or MaxTRAQ, you can calculate the angle of takeoff and the initial resultant velocity. You can then use those numbers to solve for the calculations in the individual laboratory report. If your lab is not equipped with this software, you can use the following hypothetical data to solve for these variables:

A ball is kicked with a resultant velocity of 21 m/s at an angle 32° counterclockwise from the horizontal.

Question Set 5.2

Using the data from kickers 1 and 2 on the individual laboratory report, answer the following questions:

1. Calculate the initial x velocity of the soccer ball for both kicks.
   a. Kick 1: _____
   b. Kick 2: _____
2. Calculate the initial y velocity of the soccer ball for both kicks.
   a. Kick 1: _____
   b. Kick 2: _____
3. Calculate how long the ball would be in the air (time) for both kicks.
   a. Kick 1: _____
   b. Kick 2: _____

4. Calculate how far the ball would travel in the x direction (range) for both kicks.

    a. Kick 1: _____

    b. Kick 2: _____

5. Calculate the maximum height of the ball for both kicks.

    a. Kick 1: _____

    b. Kick 2: _____

LABORATORY ACTIVITY 5.2

INDIVIDUAL LABORATORY REPORTT

Name or ID number: _____ Date: _____

Tester: _____ Time: _____

Your lab instructors will provide you with the data from these two kicks to use to complete your assignment.

Data for the resultant velocity and angle of takeoff from soccer kick 1 and soccer kick 2.

	Resultant velocity (m/s)	Angle of kick
Kicker 1		
Kicker 2		

From J. Garner, C. Allen, H. Chander, and A. Knight, *Applied Biomechanics Laboratory Manual.* (Champaign, IL: Human Kinetics, 2023).

Projectile Motion: Expanding on Earlier Principles

Objectives

- Learn to solve for the horizontal component of velocity, the vertical component of velocity, the resultant velocity, and the angle of takeoff if we know the range and time a projectile is in the air.
- Learn to solve for the range, maximum height, final resultant velocity, and angle of landing if the height of takeoff or release is higher than the landing height.
- Learn to solve for the range, maximum height, final resultant velocity, and angle of landing if the height of takeoff or release is lower than the landing height.

DEFINITIONS

maximum height (in m)—The height the person or ball or travels from the ground to the apex; calculated as $\Delta^y p = {}^y v^2/2a$; in other words, to calculate the maximum height, you square the initial y velocity and then divide by 2 times acceleration due to gravity.

projectile—Any airborne body that is only subjected to gravity and wind resistance after it has left the ground.

range (in m)—How far the projectile (such as a person or ball) travels. It is calculated using this formula: $\Delta^x p = {}^x vt$; in other words, to calculate the range, you multiply the x velocity by the total time the projectile is in the air.

trajectory—The path of a projectile. This will be in the shape of a parabola.

In the laboratory for chapter 5, we learned how to solve for the range and maximum height of a projectile if we know the resultant velocity and the angle of takeoff. It's not always possible to know the resultant velocity and angle of takeoff, but by measuring the range of a projectile and the time the projectile is in the air, we can work back to solve for the horizontal (x) component of velocity, the vertical (y) component of velocity, the resultant velocity, and the angle of takeoff. We will use the same equations, but in a different order.

$\Delta p = v_i t + 1/2at^2$ (this can be used for either horizontal or vertical position)

$$v_f = v_i + at; \text{ or } t = (v_f - v_i) / a$$

$$v_f^2 = v_i^2 + 2a\Delta p$$

$$i = \text{initial}; f = \text{final}$$

We will begin this laboratory by measuring the distance (range) of a person's broad (long) jump and timing the jump from takeoff to landing. If we know the range and time, we can solve for the x component of velocity. Since we know time and vertical acceleration, we can solve for the y component of velocity. We can then use the Pythagorean theorem to solve for the resultant velocity and use the inverse tangent function to solve for the angle of takeoff.

The same rules that we learned previously apply:

1. Gravity acts in the negative vertical (y) direction. The acceleration due to gravity is -9.81 m/s^2. Gravity will reduce the vertical velocity of a person or object as it travels up towards the apex (highest point of the trajectory) until it is 0 m/s at the apex. As the person or object travels toward the ground, gravity will increase its vertical velocity in the negative direction until it is equal to the person's vertical velocity at takeoff. For example, if a person's initial y velocity is 7 m/s, their y velocity at the apex will be 0 m/s, and the person's finial y velocity right before landing will be -7 m/s.

2. Since gravity only acts in the vertical direction, there is no acceleration of the person or object in the horizontal direction ($^xa = 0$ m/s^2). This means the horizontal, or x, velocity of the person or object is constant throughout the entire trajectory. For example, if a person jumps with an initial x velocity of 4 m/s, his or her x velocity will be 4 m/s at any point along the trajectory.

3. When solving for range, since the acceleration in the x direction is 0 m/s^2, you can use the equation $\Delta p = v_i t$ (range $= x$ velocity multiplied by total time).

4. The time it takes a person or object to travel from the ground to the apex is the same amount of time it takes the person or object to travel from the apex back to the ground (time up is equal to time down).

5. When solving for time, only use the velocities in the vertical (y) direction and the acceleration in the vertical (y) direction. The acceleration in the vertical (y) direction will always be -9.81 m/s^2.

Broad Jump

Equipment

- Tape measure
- Stopwatch
- Individual laboratory report

Resultant Velocity and Angle of Takeoff

For this portion of the lab, you are going to measure and time a classmate's broad (horizontal) jump. You will be measuring the range of the jump and the time the person is in the air. Then you will work to solve for the x and y components of velocity, the resultant velocity, and the angle of takeoff.

Step 1: Choose two student volunteers to jump so data can be obtained for use in the laboratory report. Both students will be asked to perform a broad jump.

Step 2: Choose two student volunteers to measure the jump.

Step 3: Choose two student volunteers to time the jump.

Step 4: A person performs a broad jump with a range of 1.55 m in 0.56 s. Solve for the x component of velocity, the y component of velocity, the resultant velocity, and the angle of takeoff.

Step 5: Since we know the range of the jump, we can use the equation $\Delta p = {}^{x}vt$ to solve for the x component of velocity: $1.55 \text{ m} = {}^{x}v(0.56 \text{ s})$. Divide both sides by 0.56 s to solve for the x component of velocity: $(1.55 \text{ m} / 0.56 \text{ s}) = {}^{x}v$; ${}^{x}v = 2.77 \text{ m/s}$.

Step 6: Since we know the time the person was in the air ($t = 0.56$ s), we can solve for the y component of velocity using the equation: $v_f = v_i + at$. In order to use this equation, we need solve for the final velocity at the end of the jump. If we solve for the final vertical velocity, then we also know the initial vertical velocity (final y velocity is equal to initial y velocity, but the signs are opposite). So, we are going to go from point B of the parabola (the apex), where the vertical velocity is 0 m/s, to point C, at the bottom of the jump. Since this is only half the trajectory, we need to divide our time variable by 2 (0.56 s/2), so the time from point B to point C is 0.28 s. We know that acceleration in the vertical direction is -9.81 m/s^2; we can now plug the numbers into the equation: $v_f = v_i + at$; $v_f = 0 \text{ m/s} + (-9.81 \text{ m/s}^2)(0.28 \text{ s})$; $v_f = -0.75 \text{ m/s}$. If our final vertical velocity is -2.75 m/s, then our initial vertical velocity is 2.75 m/s.

Step 7: We will use the Pythagorean theorem to solve for the resultant velocity: ${}^{x}v^2 + {}^{y}v^2 = {}^{r}v^2$. If we plug our numbers into the equation, then $(2.77 \text{ m/s})^2 + (2.75 \text{ m/s})^2 = {}^{r}v^2$, so ${}^{r}v = 3.90 \text{ m/s}$. Figure 6.1 demonstrates how the x component of velocity, the y component of velocity, and the resultant velocity form a right triangle, which allows us to use the Pythagorean theorem.

Step 8: To solve for the angle of takeoff, we can take the inverse tangent of the opposite side of the triangle, which is the vertical velocity, divided by the adjacent side of the triangle, which is the horizontal velocity: $\mu = \tan^{-1}(2.75/2.77) = 44.79°$. So, the person jumped with a resultant velocity of 3.90 m/s at an angle 44.79° counterclockwise from the ground.

Here are some practice problems to work in the laboratory:

A person jumps with a range of 1.61 m with a time of 0.60 s. Solve for the following:

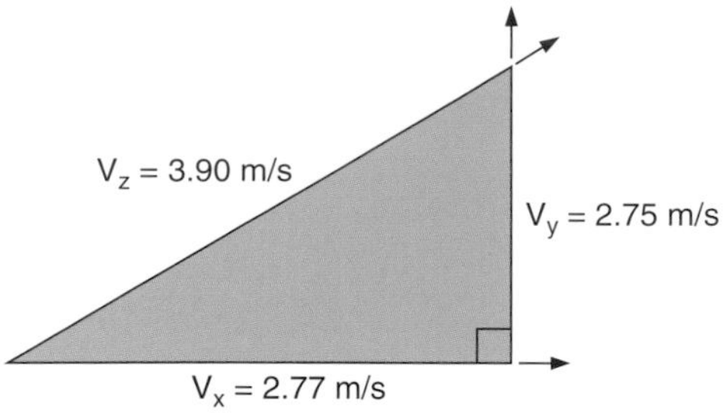

Figure 6.1 The x component, y component, and resultant velocity for the example problem.

1. The x component of velocity
2. The y component of velocity
3. The resultant velocity
4. The angle of takeoff

A person jumps with a range of 1.42 m with a time of 0.52 s. Solve for the following:

1. The x component of velocity
2. The y component of velocity
3. The resultant velocity
4. The angle of takeoff

Question Set 6.1

Using the data from jumpers 1 and 2 on the individual laboratory report for laboratory activity 6.1, answer the following questions:

1. Calculate the initial x velocity of the jumper for both jumps.
   a. Jump 1: _____
   b. Jump 2: _____
2. Calculate the initial and final y velocity of the jumper for both jumps.
   a. Jump 1: _____
   b. Jump 2: _____
3. Calculate the resultant velocity for both jumps.
   a. Jump 1: _____
   b. Jump 2: _____
4. Calculate the angle of takeoff for both jumps.
   a. Jump 1: _____
   b. Jump 2: _____

Jumping Off a Box

Equipment

- Tape measure
- Box
- Video camera or smartphone
- Individual laboratory report

Resultant Velocity and Angle of Takeoff From Jumping Off a Box

For this activity, we are going to solve for the range, maximum height, final resultant velocity, and angle at landing for a projectile that lands at a lower height than it was projected from. An example would be a person jumping down from a box. We will use the same equations we have used previously. The steps are similar to

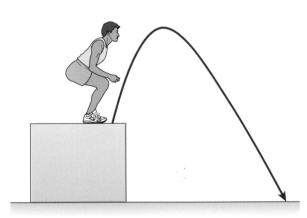

what we learned in laboratory activity 6.1, but because the person is going to be in the air longer coming down from the apex, there is an additional step that must be performed to calculate the final vertical velocity before solving for time. Then you can solve for the range, maximum height, final resultant velocity, and angle of landing. Figure 6.2 illustrates the problem we are working.

For this portion, you will need to measure the height of a box a participant will jump off of and calculate the participant's angle of takeoff and initial resultant velocity. A sample problem is given below.

Figure 6.2   Trajectory of a person jumping off a box.

A person jumps off a 1.2 m high box with an initial resultant velocity of 4 m/s at an angle 56° counterclockwise from the ground. Solve for the person's range, maximum height, final resultant velocity, and angle at landing.

Step 1: Choose two student volunteers to jump off a box onto the ground.

Step 2: Choose one person to measure the height of the box.

This lab activity is accompanied by a video demonstration on HK*Propel*.

www

Step 3: Choose one person to record the jump. If you have video analysis software, you can determine the angle of takeoff and initial resultant velocity.

Step 4: Take the resultant velocity and angle and solve for the x and y components of the resultant velocity. This is where you will use the sine and cosine functions.

$$x \text{ velocity: } \cos 56° \ (4 \text{ m/s}) = 2.24 \text{ m/s}$$

$$y \text{ velocity: } \sin 56° \ (4 \text{ m/s}) = 3.32 \text{ m/s}$$

In this example, the x velocity is adjacent to the angle, and the y velocity is opposite. That is why we are using the cosine function to solve for the x velocity and the sine function to solve for the y velocity. Since we have an angle of 56°, the y velocity should be larger than the x velocity.

Step 5:   Solve for the final y velocity, using the equation $v_f^2 = v_i^2 + 2a\Delta p$. If we make our initial y velocity the velocity of the person when they reach the same height coming down that they started at (the height of the box), then we know the following variables: the initial y velocity is equal to −3.32 m/s, acceleration is equal to −9.81 m/s², and the vertical displacement (Δp) is −1.2 m (the height of the box). We can then plug these numbers into the equation: $v_f^2 = (−3.32$ m/s$)^2 + 2(−9.81$ m/s²$)(−1.2$ m$)$. If we perform the math, we get $v_f^2 = 34.57$ m²/s², and then we need to take the square root of both sides of the equation, so we are left with $v_f = 5.88$ m/s. Since the person is moving down at this point toward the ground, this would be a negative number, so the final y velocity would be equal to −5.88 m/s.

Step 6:   Solve for time. When solving for time, you only use the velocities and accelerations in the y (vertical) direction. We know that for a projectile motion problem, the acceleration in the vertical direction will always be −9.81 m/s². We solved for the initial y velocity in step 4, and we solved for the final y velocity in step 5. We just need to plug these numbers into the equation for time. To solve for time, we use the equation $t = (v_f − v_i)/a$. Again, when solving for time, we only use the velocities and acceleration in the vertical direction. We know that the final y velocity is −5.88 m/s, the initial y velocity is 3.32 m/s, and the acceleration is −9.81 m/s². We just need to plug these numbers into our equation: $t = (−5.88$ m/s $− 3.32$ m/s$)/−9.81$ m/s². By doing the math, we determine that time = 0.94 s.

Step 7:   Now we can solve for range. The range is the horizontal (x) displacement. We can use the equation $\Delta p = v_i t + \frac{1}{2}at^2$. Since the acceleration in the horizontal direction is 0 m/s² (remember, gravity only acts in the vertical direction), we can simplify this equation to read $\Delta p = v_i t$. Since this is horizontal displacement, we have to use our initial x velocity, which is 2.24 m/s. We just need to multiply this velocity by time to solve for the range:

$$\Delta^x p = (2.24 \text{ m/s})(0.94 \text{ s}) = 2.11 \text{ m}$$

This tells us the person traveled 2.11 m in the horizontal direction from the top of the box to the ground.

Step 8:   The next thing to solve for is the maximum height, or height of the person or object from the ground at the apex. In this type of problem, we can either solve for the vertical displacement from the top of the box or the apex, or we can solve for the vertical displacement from the ground to the apex.

If we choose to solve for the vertical displacement from the top of the box to the apex, we will use the same process that we used in the previous projectile motion problem from laboratory 5. We are interested in the vertical displacement from the top of the box to the apex. The simplest way to work this step is to use this equation: $v_f^2 = v_i^2 + 2a\Delta p$. Since we are in the vertical direction again, we have to go back to our vertical velocities and vertical acceleration. We are going from the top of the box to the apex, so the final vertical velocity is still 0 m/s (at the apex). We calculated the initial vertical velocity in step 4; it was 3.32 m/s, and the acceleration in the vertical direction is −9.81 m/s² (due to gravity). Since our final velocity is 0 m/s (vertical velocity at the apex), we can rearrange this equation to read that maximum height is equal to the initial y velocity squared divided by 2 times the acceleration due to gravity. Looking at the following equation, we see that h is our maximum height (vertical displacement from the ground to the apex), $^y v$ is our initial y velocity, and a is the acceleration due to gravity.

$$h = \frac{^y v^2}{a_g 2}$$

In our example, h = (3.32 m/s)² / (2*−9.81 m/s²), so h = 0.17 m.

The maximum height of the person at the apex is 0.56 m from the top of the box. Since we know the top of the box is 1.2 m from the ground, we can add this height to 0.56 m, and the vertical displacement from the apex to the ground is 1.76 m.

The other way to work this problem is to directly solve for the vertical displacement from the apex to the ground. In this case, we will use the equation $v_f^2 = v_i^2 + 2a\Delta p$. We calculated the final vertical velocity in step 5, it was −5.88 m/s. The initial vertical velocity is the velocity at the apex, which is 0 m/s. Acceleration in the vertical direction is always −9.81 m/s². We can plug these numbers into the equation to get (−5.88 m/s)² = (0 m/s)² − 2(−9.81 m/s²)(Δp). This gives us 34.57 m²/s² = 0 m²/s² −19.62 m/s²(Δp). If we then divide both sides of the equation by −19.62 m/s², we get (34.57 m²/s²/−19.62 m/s²) = Δp, which gives us Δp = −1.76 m. In this case, vertical displacement is a negative number because the person is moving from the apex toward the ground in the negative vertical direction.

Step 9:   The next step is to solve for the person's final resultant velocity. Since the person's final vertical velocity is greater than their initial vertical velocity, their final resultant velocity will be different than their initial resultant velocity. Using the Pythagorean theorem ($a^2 + b^2 = c^2$), where c represents the resultant velocity, and a and b represent the horizontal and vertical components of velocity, we can solve for the final resultant velocity. The horizontal velocity of the person, calculated in step 4, is 2.24 m/s, and the final vertical velocity of the person, calculated in step 5, is −5.88 m/s. We just need to plug these numbers into the Pythagorean theorem: (2.24 m/s)² + −5.88 m/s² = c^2; 39.59 m²/s² = c^2. If we take the square root of 39.59 m²/s², we get 6.29 m/s. This is the final resultant velocity of the person. If you notice, this velocity is greater than their initial resultant velocity of 4 m/s, because the person's final vertical velocity is greater than their initial vertical velocity.

Step 10:   The last step is to solve for the angle at which the person contacts the ground. If we construct a right angle with the components and resultant velocity, we can use the inverse tangent function to solve for the angle (much like we did in our previous problem). Tangent is the ratio of the opposite side over the adjacent side. In our problem, the opposite side is the horizontal component of velocity (2.24 m/s), and the adjacent side is the vertical component of the velocity vector (−5.88 m/s). Mathematically, we would take the $\tan^{-1}$ (2.24/−5.88), which will give us −20.85°.

Question Set 6.2

Using the data from jumpers 1 and 2 on the individual laboratory report for laboratory activity 6.2, answer the following questions:

1. Calculate the initial x velocity and initial y velocity of the jump.
   a. Initial x velocity: _____
   b. Initial y velocity: _____
2. Calculate the final y velocity of the jump.
   a. Final y velocity: _____
3. Solve for the time the person is in the air.
   a. Time: _____
4. Solve for the range of the person.
   a. Range: _____
5. Solve for the maximum height of the person.
   a. Maximum height from the top of the box to the apex: _____
   b. Maximum height from the ground to the apex: _____
6. Solve for the final resultant velocity of the person.
   a. Final resultant velocity: _____
7. Solve for the angle of landing.
   a. Angle: _____

Jumping Up Onto a Box

Equipment

- Tape measure
- Video camera or smartphone
- Box
- Individual laboratory report

Resultant Velocity and Angle of Takeoff From Jumping Onto a Box

In this activity, we are going to solve for the range, maximum height, final resultant velocity, and angle at landing for a projectile that lands at a higher height than it was projected from. An example would be a person jumping up onto a box. We will use the same equations we have used previously. The steps are similar to what we learned in the previous problem, but because the person is going to be in the air a lesser amount of time coming down from the apex, there is an additional step that must be performed to calculate the final vertical velocity before solving for time. Then, you can solve for the range, maximum height, final resultant velocity, and angle of landing. Figure 6.3 illustrates this movement.

For this portion, you will need to measure the height of a box a participant will jump up onto and calculate the participant's angle of takeoff and initial resultant velocity. A sample problem is given below.

A person jumps up onto a 0.9 m high box with an initial resultant velocity of 5 m/s at an angle 66° CCW from the ground. Solve for the person's range, maximum height, final resultant velocity, and angle at landing.

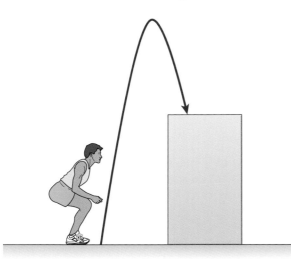

Figure 6.3 Trajectory of a person jumping up onto a box.

Step 1: Choose two student volunteers to jump up onto a box from the ground.

> This lab is accompanied by a video demonstration on HK*Propel*.
>
> www

Step 2: Choose one student volunteer to measure the height of the box.

Step 3: Choose one student volunteer to record the jump. If you have video analysis software, you can determine the angle of takeoff and initial resultant velocity.

Step 4: Take the resultant velocity and angle and solve for the x and y components of the resultant velocity. This is where you will use the sine and cosine functions.

$$x \text{ velocity: } \cos 66° (5 \text{ m/s}) = 2.03 \text{ m/s}$$

$$y \text{ velocity: } \sin 66° (5 \text{ m/s}) = 4.57 \text{ m/s}$$

In this example, the x velocity is adjacent to the angle, and the y velocity is opposite. That is why we are using the cosine function to solve for the x velocity and the sine function to solve for the y velocity. Since we have an angle of 66°, the y velocity should be larger than the x velocity.

Step 5:   Before we can solve for time, we need to solve for the final y velocity. However, before we can do this, we need to solve for the maximum height of the jump (from the ground to the apex), and then subtract the height of the box from this value. This will give us the person's vertical displacement from the apex to the top of the box. In this step, we are going from the ground to the apex of the jump. This means the person's final vertical velocity will be 0 m/s. The person's initial vertical velocity was calculated in step 4, and it is 4.57 m/s. Acceleration in the vertical direction is −9.81 m/s². We will use the equation: $v_f^2 = v_i^2 + 2a\Delta p$, and we can rearrange this equation to read that maximum height is equal to the initial y velocity squared divided by 2 times the acceleration due to gravity. Looking at the equation below, we see that h is our maximum height (vertical displacement from the ground to the apex), $^y v$ is our initial y velocity, and a_g is the acceleration due to gravity.

$$h = \frac{^y v^2}{a_g 2}$$

In our example, $h = (4.57 \text{ m/s})^2/(2\star{-}9.81 \text{ m/s}^2)$, so $h = 1.06$ m.

The maximum height of the person at the apex is 1.06 m from the top of the ground. To solve for the person's final vertical velocity in the next step, we need to know the person's displacement from the apex to the top of the box. The height of the box is 0.9 m, and the height of the person at the apex of the jump is 1.06 m. If we subtract 0.9 m from 1.06 m (1.06 m − 0.9 m), the person's vertical displacement from the apex to the top of the box is 0.16 m. We will use this value in our next step.

Step 6:   Solve for the final y velocity (right before the person lands on the box), using the equation $v_f^2 = v_i^2 + 2a\Delta p$. Our initial y velocity will be the person's velocity at the apex of the jump, which is 0 m/s. The person's vertical displacement is −0.16 m (negative because they are moving down in the negative vertical direction), and the acceleration in the vertical direction is −9.81 m/s², due to gravity. We can then plug these numbers into the equation: $v_f^2 = (0 \text{ m/s})^2 + 2(-9.81 \text{ m/s}^2)(-0.16 \text{ m})$. If we perform the math, we get $v_f^2 = 3.14 \text{ m}^2/\text{s}^2$, and then we need to take the square root of both sides of the equation, so we are left with $v_f = 1.77$ m/s. Since the person is moving down at this point towards the ground, this would be a negative number, so the final y velocity would be equal to −1.77 m/s.

Step 7:   Solve for time. When solving for time, you only use the velocities and accelerations in the y (vertical) direction. We know that for a projectile motion problem the acceleration in the vertical direction will always be −9.81 m/s². We solved for the initial y velocity in step 1, and we solved for the final y velocity in step 3. We just need to plug these numbers into the equation for time. To solve for time, we use the equation $t = (v_f - v_i) / a$. Again, when solving for time we only use the velocities and acceleration in the vertical direction. We know that the final y velocity is -1.77 m/s, the initial y velocity is 4.47 m/s, and acceleration is -9.81 m/s². We just need to plug these numbers into our equation: $t = (-1.77$ m/s $- 4.57$ m/s$)/-9.81$ m/s². By doing the math, we find that time = 0.65 s.

Step 8: Now we can solve for range. The range is the horizontal (x) displacement, which in this example would be how far the person jumped to land on the box. We can use the equation $\Delta p = v_i t + 1/2at^2$. Since the acceleration in the horizontal direction is 0 m/s² (remember, gravity only acts in the vertical direction), we can simplify this equation to read $\Delta p = v_i t$. Since this is horizontal displacement, we have to use our initial x velocity, which is 2.24 m/s. We just need to multiply this velocity by time to solve for the range:

$$\Delta^x p = (2.03 \text{ m/s})(0.65 \text{ s}) = 1.32 \text{ m}$$

This tells us the person traveled 1.32 m in the horizontal direction from the ground to the top of the box.

Step 9: The next step is to solve for the person's final resultant velocity. Since the person's final vertical velocity is less than their initial vertical velocity, their final resultant velocity will be different (less) than their initial resultant velocity. Using the Pythagorean theorem ($a^2 + b^2 = c^2$), where c represents the resultant velocity, and a and b represent the horizontal and vertical components of velocity, we can solve for the final resultant velocity. The horizontal velocity of the person, calculated in step 1, is 2.03 m/s, and the final vertical velocity of the person, calculated in step 2, is -1.77 m/s. We just need to plug these numbers into the Pythagorean theorem: $(2.03 \text{ m/s})^2 + (-1.77 \text{ m/s})^2 = c^2$; $7.25 \text{ m}^2/\text{s}^2 = c^2$. If we take the square root of 7.25 m²/s², we get 2.69 m/s. This is the final resultant velocity of the person. If you notice, this velocity is less than their initial resultant velocity of 5 m/s, because the person's final vertical velocity is less than their initial vertical velocity.

Step 10: The last step is to solve for the angle at which the person contacts the ground. If we construct a right angle with the components and resultant velocity, we can use the inverse tangent function to solve for the angle (much like we did in our previous problem). Tangent is the ratio of the opposite side over the adjacent side. In our problem, the opposite side is the horizontal component of velocity (2.03 m/s), and the adjacent side is the vertical component of the velocity vector (-1.77 m/s). Mathematically, we would take the $\tan^{-1}(2.03/-1.77)$, which will give us $-48.91°$.

Question Set 6.3

Using the data from jumpers 1 and 2 on the individual laboratory report, answer the following questions:

1. Calculate the initial x velocity and initial y velocity of the jump.
   a. Initial x velocity: _____
   b. Initial y velocity: _____

2. Solve for the maximum height of the person.

    a. Maximum height from the ground to the apex of the jump: _____

    b. Vertical displacement from the apex of the jump to the top of the box: _____

3. Calculate the final y velocity of the jump.

    a. Final y velocity: _____

4. Solve for the time the person is in the air.

    a. Time: _____

5. Solve for the range of the person.

    a. Range: _____

6. Solve for the final resultant velocity of the person.

    a. Final resultant velocity: _____

7. Solve for the angle of landing.

    a. Angle: _____

INDIVIDUAL LABORATORY REPORT

Name or ID number: _____ Date: _____

Tester: _____ Time: _____

Laboratory Activity 6.1

You will have the data for your lab report before you leave the lab.

Data for the resultant velocity and angle of takeoff from jumper 1 and jumper 2.

	Range (m)	Time (s)
Jumper 1		
Jumper 2		

Always measure distance in cm if possible. 100 cm = 1 m. If you measure the distance in inches, then you will need to convert it into cm; 1 inch = 2.54 cm.

Laboratory Activity 6.2

You will have the data for your lab report before you leave the lab.

Data for the resultant velocity and angle of takeoff from jumping off a box.

	Height of box (m)	Angle of takeoff (degrees)	Resultant velocity (m/s)
Jumper 1			
Jumper 2			
Example data	0.8 m	62°	4.4 m/s

Laboratory Activity 6.3

You will have the data for your lab report before you leave the lab.

Data for the resultant velocity and angle of takeoff from jumping onto a box.

	Height of box (m)	Angle of takeoff (degrees)	Resultant velocity (m/s)
Jumper 1			
Jumper 1			
Example data	0.8 m	62°	4.4 m/s

From J. Garner, C. Allen, H. Chander, and A. Knight, *Applied Biomechanics Laboratory Manual.* (Champaign, IL: Human Kinetics, 2023).

Angular Kinematics

Objectives

- Demonstrate an understanding of angular kinematics.
- Apply the principles of angular kinematics to sport performance, ergonomics, and injury rehabilitation.

DEFINITIONS

angle (μ)—A figure formed by the intersection of two planes, two lines, or a line and a plane. Typically, the symbol μ represents the angle or angular position. An angle can be measured in both degrees and radians, where 1 rad = 57.3°.

angular position (μ)—The orientation of a line or plane in reference to another line or plane. Depending on the object of interest, the joint involved, or the activity, angular position can be measured with various forms of technology ranging from a simple goniometer to a sophisticated motion-capture system. Angular position can be measured in both degrees and radians, where 1 rad = 57.3°.

angular displacement (Δμ)—The rotational change in the orientation of an object.

angular velocity (ω)—The rate of the rotational change in the orientation of an object or the rate of change of the angular displacement. This can also be defined as how fast an object is rotating in a particular direction.

angular acceleration (α)—The rate at which an object's angular velocity is changing in a particular direction. This can also be defined as how quickly an object is speeding up or slowing down its rotation in a particular direction.

CALCULATING ANGULAR KINEMATICS

Angular Displacement

Much like linear displacement, we must know several factors to properly measure or calculate angular displacement. These factors include:

- **axis of rotation**—The point about which the circular motion occurs. Examples of the axis rotation could include the joint center for limb movements, or the body's center of mass when performing a flip. Although the axis of rotation is not directly used in the angular displacement calculation, it is vital to know the point about which the motion occurs.
- **final angular position**—The final point of the movement of interest, often referred to as μ_f.
- **initial angular position**—The beginning point of the movement of interest, often referred to as μ_i.

Angular displacement is calculated by determining the difference between the object's final angular position and its initial angular position.

$$\Delta\mu = \mu_f - \mu_i$$

Angular displacement can be measured in both degrees and radians, where 1 rad = 57.3°.

Calculating Angular Velocity

In order to calculate angular velocity, we must be able to determine several components:

- **final angular position**—The final point of the movement of interest, often referred to as μ_f
- **initial angular position**—The beginning point of the movement of interest, often referred to as μ_i

- **time**—The time taken for the motion of interest to occur, referred as Δt or t.

Angular velocity is calculated by dividing the difference between the object's final angular position and its initial angular position by the time it took to move between those positions. More simply, it is the change in angular position divided by time.

$$\varpi = \frac{\Delta \theta}{\Delta t} = \frac{\theta_f - \theta_i}{\Delta t}$$

The most common units of measure for angular velocity include radians per second (rad/s), degrees per second (°/s), and revolutions per minute (rpm).

Angular acceleration is calculated by dividing the difference between the object's final angular velocity and its initial angular velocity by the time it took to move between those velocities. More simply, it is the change in angular velocity divided by time.

$$\alpha = \frac{\delta \omega}{\delta t} = \frac{\omega_f - \omega_i}{\delta t}$$

The most common units of measure for angular acceleration include radians per second per second (rad/s/s or rad/s²), degrees per second per second (°/s/s or °/s²), or any other angular acceleration per unit time.

RELATING ANGULAR KINEMATICS TO LINEAR KINEMATICS

While angular motion is a critical aspect of human movement, it is also important to identify the linear speed of an object or segment that is rotating. This might include a baseball or softball bat, a tennis racquet, or the distal end of a segment, such as the hand during the throwing motion or the foot during the kicking motion. In order to calculate the linear velocity of a rotating segment, two things must be known:

1. The angular velocity of the rigid body (υ)
2. The distance from the point on the rigid body to the axis of rotation (l_r), referred to as the length of the radius

The linear velocity of a point on a rotating segment is calculated by multiplying the angular velocity of the segment by the length of the radius.

$$v = l \times \upsilon$$

Angular velocity should be in rad/s to make this calculation. The units of measurement are m/s. This equation demonstrates that in order to increase the linear velocity of a point on a rotating segment, you can increase angular velocity, the length of the radius, or both. Examples of this are readily available across the landscape of sport and occupational settings. Although swinging a golf club and sledgehammer seem to be vastly different, the goal of delivering the head of the implement with maximal velocity remains the same. To get the most bang out of the effort, the athlete or worker will often choose the longest club or tool they can control. By swinging a slightly longer implement with the same angular velocity, they are able to generate the most linear velocity of the implement's head at the moment of impact.

UNDERSTANDING ANGULAR KINEMATICS

Unlike linear kinematics, where all points move in a straight line, angular kinematics deal with situations where all points on an object move in circular motion. The ability to understand and apply the principles of angular kinematics is a vital skill within the realm of human movement. Almost every motion of humans, and other animals, for that matter, relies on angular motions of the limbs around fixed joints to produce movement. Although they may appear very different at first glance, the principles of angular kinematics are very similar to those of linear kinematics.

Angular Kinematic Applications to Sport Performance

Proper angular kinematics is important for safe, effective, and appropriate movement during sport and physical activity. Proper angular displacement, across joints in the kinetic or kinematic chain is not only necessary for performance, but also to reduce injury risk. For example, adequate ankle dorsiflexion during closed-chain exercises such as the back squat allows greater anterior knee movement, which results in a trunk angle closer to vertical. Conversely, a lack of ankle dorsiflexion limits forward knee movement, which increases lumbar spinal flexion (List et al., 2013), resulting in increased spinal loading (Fry et al., 2003; Whitting et al., 2016) particularly in novice lifters.

Angular velocity and acceleration are also important factors in sport performance. Examples come from sports involving throwing or hitting a ball such as baseball, softball, and tennis. Throwing or hitting activities involve rotationally accelerating body segments in a sequential manner with the goal of achieving maximal rotational velocity and transferring energy and momentum to the ball. As the throw or swing is initiated, this sequential rotation occurs in a proximal to distal fashion beginning with the pelvis, trunk, arms, hands, and finally the bat or ball (Putnam, 1983). The larger, more proximal body segments (pelvis and trunk) accelerate achieving relatively slow rotational velocities, but as these segments begin to slow down, the smaller, more distal segments (arms and hands) accelerate, achieving faster rotational velocities (Escamilla et al., 2009; Fleisig et al., 1999).

In addition to speeding up the rotation of body segments, athletes also need to be able to slow down and stop this motion as well, particularly during activities requiring agility and change of direction. This could be as part of a preplanned movement such as a wide receiver running a pass route in American football, or in response to a stimulus such as a soccer defender changing their running speed and direction as the result of their opponent's movement. In both cases, the athletes must slow down (negatively accelerate) the rotation of their leg segments, reorient their bodies, and quickly reaccelerate in the desired movement direction.

Angular Kinematic Applications to Injury and Rehabilitation

Injuries commonly occur when the angular displacement of a segment exceeds the normal anatomical limits, typically with a high angular velocity. For example, the lateral ankle sprain, which is one of the most frequently occurring injuries in sports (Herzog et al., 2019), typically occurs with a combination of excessive inversion and internal rotation of the rear foot. A lateral ankle sprain that was recently recorded in a laboratory setting occurred with a combination of 55° of inversion and 27° of internal rotation, with an inversion angular velocity of 927°/s (Li et al., 2019). This large amount of angular displacement and high angular velocity places excessive stress on the lateral ankle ligaments, leading to injury (Hertel, 2019).

Preventing excessive angular displacement at a joint can help lower the risk of a ligamentous injury. Eccentric muscle actions can provide some protection against these potential injury mechanisms (Konradsen et al., 1997). Bracing and taping is another mechanism that can be used to limit the amount of angular displacement and reduce the angular velocity at a joint, and thus lower the risk of injury (Papadopoulos et al., 2005). Knowledge of the normal range of motion at each joint can help a practitioner examine patients and athletes and determine their injury risk. Patients or athletes who have an increased amount of angular displacement or range of motion at a joint would have an increased risk of injury. Range of motion measurements obtained through the use of a goniometer can be useful for assessing changes in range of motion that may occur over time, such as after an injury. These measurements can also be useful for comparing the range of motion at joints on contralateral sides of the body.

Angular Kinematic Applications to Human Factors and Ergonomics

Measurement of human body kinematics at various joints of the upper and lower extremities including the spine, during different occupational tasks aid in understanding the injury risk of each occupational task and subsequently to make work-task modifications or to train in order to improve performance and safety. Work-related musculoskeletal disorders, which include a wide range of inflammatory and degenerative conditions, are a common occurrence in multiple industries and occupations (Punnett & Wegman, 2004), especially in construction, manufacturing, and warehousing, where there is more exposure to manual material handling. Extremes of joint range of motion, rapid and repetitive movements, improper manual material handling techniques, nonneutral static, and dynamic postures and overexertion (Kumar, 1999; Punnett & Wegman, 2004) are all factors contributing to work-related musculoskeletal disorders. As such, kinematic analysis of whole-body or specific-body segments to include more than one joint or specific individual joints can prove to be very valuable in human factors and ergonomics.

Kumar (1999) proposed an empirical relationship between the job range of motion and the job-mediated risk of overexertion injuries. Even though the exact joint range of motion in which there is a greater mechanical and physiological advantage can vary based on the joint and movement performed, the extremes of range of motion have the greatest mechanical and physiological disadvantage (Kumar, 1999). The midrange position is designated as the risk neutral zone as it perceived to be of low risk and comfortable and requires a minimal, efficient effort for performing the work task. Deviations from the risk-neutral midrange increases the job-mediated risk and is considered hazardous to the worker (Kumar, 1999).

The nature and the environment of the job dictates the type of methods used for kinematic measurements in human factors and ergonomics. Methods for measuring kinematics in occupational settings include simple and advanced observational techniques (David, 2005). Some examples of simple observational methods for assessing static and dynamic postures and kinematics include the Ovako working posture assessment system, rapid upper limb assessment, and rapid entire-body assessment (David, 2005). More advanced observational methods include the use of a simple goniometer, electric goniometer, accelerometers, inertial measurement units, inclinometers, and 2D and 3D video motion-capture analysis (David, 2005).

An example of kinematic measurement in human ergonomics is the military load carriage task. This physically demanding, strenuous task is associated with multiple aspects of acute musculoskeletal injuries and work-related musculoskeletal disorders. As such, military load carriage can significantly influence lower extremity kinematics during gait. Three-dimensional motion-capture analysis of load carriage gait has been studied extensively and has reported changes in ankle, knee, hip, pelvis, and trunk kinematics (Attwells et al., 2006; Birrell & Haslam, 2009; Birrell & Haslam, 2010; Chander et al., 2020; Majumdar et al., 2009).

Goniometry Measurement of Joint Angles and Angular Displacement

Equipment

- Goniometer
- Examination table
- Towel or small pillow
- Individual laboratory report

Goniometry Assessment of Elbow Joint Range of Motion

Step 1: Choose a student volunteer to lie supine on the examination table with legs straight, arms at sides, and forearms supinated. It might be necessary to place a rolled-up towel or small pillow under the distal aspect of the participant's humerus to keep the shoulder in a neutral position.

Step 2: Place the fulcrum of the goniometer over the lateral epicondyle of the humerus. The stationary arm should align with the acromion process at the shoulder and approximate the long axis of the humerus.

Step 3: Have the student volunteer place the movable arm along the long axis of the radius, in line with the styloid process. Measure the amount of elbow extension of the participant. Full extension is considered to be 0°. Some individuals have an increased amount of joint laxity and might have approximately −1 to 10° of hyperextension.

Step 4: Have the participant flex the elbow through a full range of motion. Most people have approximately 145° to 150° of elbow flexion.

Step 5: Reposition the goniometer using the landmarks previously described and measure the amount of elbow flexion of the participant.

Step 6: Repeat these steps for both the left and right side and record the measurements in the appropriate section of the individual laboratory report. Figure 7.1 demonstrates this measurement.

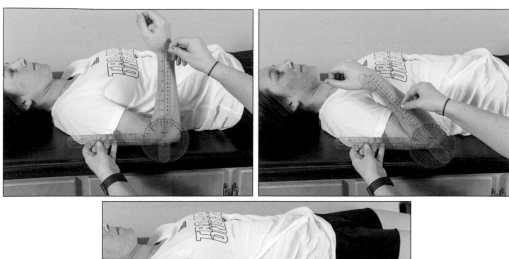

Figure 7.1 Assessing elbow joint range of motion with a goniometer.

Question Set 7.1

1. Compare the goniometry range of motion assessments you obtained to the data obtained by a classmate. What is one reason why elbow flexion range of motion would be different from individual to individual? Explain.

2. What is one reason why elbow flexion range of motion may differ from left to right side for the same individual? Explain.

Calculating Angular Velocity and Angular Acceleration

Equipment

- Smart device camera
- Dumbbell
- Individual laboratory report

2D Camera and Software Procedures to Measure Joint Angles and Angular Displacement

Note: Alternative instruments, such as a 2D video camera, alternative smart device apps, video analysis software such as Dartfish or MaxTRAQ, or a 3D motion-capture system, can be used to complete this component of the lab. Specific procedures for these alternative instruments will vary. If you are using a motion-capture system, please use the system's prescribed marker placement (clusters vs. individual markers).

While a goniometer is a good tool to measure range of motion and determine total angular displacement, for measuring and calculating angular velocity and angular acceleration, we need more advanced tools, such as a video camera and 2D motion-analysis software like Dartfish or MaxTRAQ, or a 3D motion-capture system. To measure elbow flexion and extension with a camera or motion-capture system, markers should be placed on the acromion process, lateral humeral condyle, and styloid process of the radius. The participant can then flex and extend his or her elbow while the camera or motion-capture system tracks the angular position of the forearm, which can then be used to determine angular displacement, angular velocity, and angular acceleration. Similar procedures can be used for angular kinematic measurements at other joints.

Step 1: Choose a student volunteer. On the right side of the participant's body, place reflective markers on the acromion process of the scapula, lateral humeral condyle, and radial styloid process.

Step 2: Position the smart device camera for a sagittal plane view of a participant so that all reflective markers are in view of the camera.

Step 3: Access a video analysis smart device app and prepare to record a new video.

Step 4: Instruct the volunteer participant to perform a dumbbell curl, flexing the elbow in a controlled manner through a full range of motion, and then extending the elbow in a similar fashion to return to the starting position. Total movement time should be approximately 3 seconds.

Step 5: Use the app to record the participant performing the dumbbell curl.

Step 6: Use the app tools to determine joint angle position at time intervals of 0.25 seconds and record the data appropriate section of the individual laboratory report.

Step 7: Once data has been transferred to the individual date sheet, record calculations of angular displacement, angular velocity, angular acceleration, and other variables in the appropriate section of the individual laboratory report. Figure 7.2 demonstrates this process.

> This lab is accompanied by a video demonstration in HK*Propel*.
>
> **WWW**

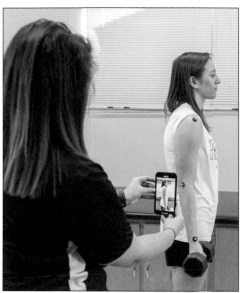
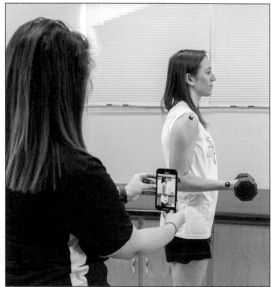
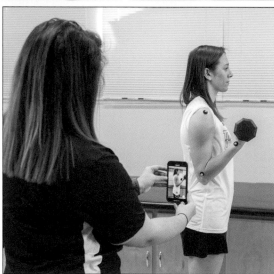

Figure 7.2 Smartphone camera setup for measuring and calculating angular velocity and angular acceleration.

Question Set 7.2

1. Why would using a 2D or 3D motion-capture device allow for more precision of measurement compared to a goniometer?

2. Discuss the positives and negatives related to a motion-capture device compared to a handheld goniometer.

Calculating Linear Velocity From Angular Velocity

Equipment

- Measuring tape
- Measured or hypothetical data calculations from laboratory activity 7.2

Procedures

Step 1: Choose a student volunteer and measure the length of the forearm and hand (in meters) of the participant (or measure a classmate's forearm and hand length if using the hypothetical data).

Step 2: Record that length in the appropriate column on the individual laboratory report. This measurement is the length of the rotating segment (radius).

Step 3: In the appropriate column, record the measured or hypothetical angular velocities in degrees per second (°/s).

Step 4: Convert the angular velocities from degrees per second (°/s) to radians per second (rad/s).

Step 5: Multiply the radius length by the angular velocity in radians per second (rad/s) at each point to determine the linear velocity of the hand at that point.

Step 6: Record those calculations in the linear velocity column on the individual laboratory report.

Question Set 7.3

1. Compare the linear and angular velocity of participants with different lower arm lengths. What was the reason their linear velocity was different than those with a similar angular velocity?

2. Why is calculating linear velocity of a rotating segment from angular velocity data a useful skill?

3. Use your answer to the previous question to explain why a major league baseball team might choose to draft a 6 ft, 6 in. (1.98 m), 17-year-old high school pitcher over a 6 ft, 1 in. (1.85 m) 22-year-old collegiate pitcher when both athletes throw a 94- to 95-mile-per-hour fastball.

INDIVIDUAL LABORATORY REPORT

Laboratory Activity 7.1   Goniometry Assessment of Elbow Joint Range of Motion

Left elbow		Right elbow	
Full extension angle		Full extension angle	
Full flexion angle		Full flexion angle	
Amount of angular displacement		Amount of angular displacement	

Laboratory Activity 7.2   Elbow Joint Sample Range of Motion Data

Point	Angular position	Time
1		0 s
2		0.25 s
3		0.5 s
4		0.75 s
5		1.0 s
6		1.25 s
7		1.50 s
8		1.75 s
9		2.0 s
10		2.25 s
11		2.50 s
12		2.75 s
13		3.0 s

From J. Garner, C. Allen, H. Chander, and A. Knight, *Applied Biomechanics Laboratory Manual.* (Champaign, IL: Human Kinetics, 2023).

Angular Kinematic Calculations From Sample Elbow Joint Data

Point	Time	Cumulative angular distance (°)	Cumulative angular displacement (°)	Interval angular distance (°)	Angular speed (°/s)	Interval angular displacement (°)	Angular velocity (°/s)	Change in angular velocity (°/s)	Angular acceleration (°/s²)
1	0 s	0°	0°	0°	0°/s	0°	0 °/s	0 °/s	0 °/s²
2	0.25 s								
3	0.5 s								
4	0.75 s								
5	1.0 s								
6	1.25 s								
7	1.50 s								
8	1.75 s								
9	2.0 s								
10	2.25 s								
11	2.50 s								
12	2.75 s								
13	3.0 s								

Use the hypothetical data in the following table if these instruments are unavailable. The participant is starting in full elbow extension (0°), moving into flexion (approximately 145°-150°), then moving back to full extension.

Elbow Joint Sample Range of Motion Data

Point	Angular position	Time
1	0°	0 s
2	32°	0.25 s
3	65°	0.5 s
4	97°	0.75 s
5	125°	1.0 s
6	147°	1.25 s
7	147°	1.50 s
8	121°	1.75 s
9	100°	2.0 s
10	74°	2.25 s
11	45°	2.50 s
12	18°	2.75 s
13	0°	3.0 s

From J. Garner, C. Allen, H. Chander, and A. Knight, *Applied Biomechanics Laboratory Manual*. (Champaign, IL: Human Kinetics, 2023).

The elbow joint data table that follows can be used to record calculations of angular displacement, angular velocity, angular acceleration, and other variables.

Angular Kinematic Calculations From Sample Elbow Joint Data

Point	Time	Cumulative angular distance (°)	Cumulative angular displacement (°)	Interval angular distance (°)	Angular speed (°/s)	Interval angular displacement (°)	Angular velocity (°/s)	Change in angular velocity (°/s)	Angular acceleration (°/s²)
1	0 s	0°	0°	0°	0°/s	0°	0 °/s	0 °/s	0 °/s²
2	0.25 s								
3	0.5 s								
4	0.75 s								
5	1.0 s								
6	1.25 s								
7	1.50 s								
8	1.75 s								
9	2.0 s								
10	2.25 s								
11	2.50 s								
12	2.75 s								
13	3.0 s								

Laboratory Activity 7.3 Calculating Linear Velocity From Angular Velocity

Point	Radius (l_r)	Angular velocity (°/s)	Angular velocity (rad/s)	Linear velocity (m/s)
1		0 °/s	0 rad/s	0 m/s
2				
3				
4				
5				
6				
7				
8				
9				
10				
11				
12				
13				

From J. Garner, C. Allen, H. Chander, and A. Knight, *Applied Biomechanics Laboratory Manual*. (Champaign, IL: Human Kinetics, 2023).

Linear Kinetics: Ground Reaction Forces

Objectives

- Understand the principles of linear kinetics.
- Apply linear kinetics to the fields of sport performance, ergonomics, and injury and rehabilitation.

DEFINITIONS

ground reaction forces—The force exerted by the ground on a body in contact with it.

Newton's first law of motion (inertia)—An object at rest or in constant motion will remain at rest or in constant motion unless acted upon by external forces. In short, inertia is an object's resistance to change in its current state of motion. This resistance can be indirectly measured by the object's mass (kg). An object with a larger mass will have a greater resistance to change in motion than an object with a smaller mass and will require a larger force to overcome that resistance. Inertia can also be defined as a resistance to acceleration.

Newton's second law of motion (acceleration)—The amount of force necessary to overcome inertia. An object's acceleration depends on two things: the object's mass and the net sum of forces applied (both magnitude and direction of application) to the object. This introduces one of the most famous equations in mechanics and can be viewed as a cause-and-effect relationship, meaning that the forces cause the change in the velocity of the mass.

$$\Sigma F = m \times a$$

- ΣF—the sum of all forces (N) acting on an object or system
- m—the mass (kg)
- a—the acceleration (m/s^2) of the object.

Newton's third law of motion (reaction)—Newton's third law of motion states that for every force, there is a second force, equal in magnitude and opposite in direction. In other words, forces occur in opposing pairs.

Kinetics is the study of the forces that cause or resist motion. In order for an object or body to move or resist movement, a force must be applied. A force is simply defined as a push or pull on an object. This force may be direct, such as picking up a box, or indirect, such as a magnet picking up a paper clip. Forces may also be classified as internal or external. Internal forces are those that act inside a system or body, such as muscles pulling on bones to generate a joint action or the compressive forces experienced by spinal vertebrae due to gravity. While these internal forces are important for the study of

injury, they do not directly cause movement. Movement is caused when the body can either push or pull against something peripheral, such as the ground or another body. This push or pull is an example of external forces that act on a body as result of contact or interaction. These external forces will be the focus of the activities in the next two labs.

Ground reaction forces are one type of external force that are frequently analyzed for activities such as walking, running, and jumping for the purposes of improving performance and decreasing injury risk. Ground reaction forces are recorded using force platforms. Force platforms are sophisticated scales with either strain gauges or transducers inside the platform for measuring force. The force platforms can be monoaxial, measuring force in a single direction (usually vertical), or triaxial, measuring force in the anterior–posterior (X) and medial–lateral (Y) dimensions in addition to the vertical (Z) dimension. These platforms can record force data at extremely high rates ranging from 100 to 1,000 Hz (data recordings per second) or higher. This force and time data can be graphed and used for more in-depth analysis (figure 8.1).

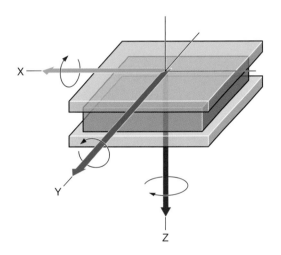

Figure 8.1 Example of a triaxial force plate.

LINEAR KINETICS APPLICATIONS TO SPORT PERFORMANCE

The countermovement vertical jump (CMVJ) is one of the most utilized assessments in sports and strength and conditioning. Requiring minimal equipment, the assessment is easily executed in a relatively small amount of time. The use of a force platform to assess CMVJ can provide insight into many aspects of performance, including force production variables, athlete readiness and fatigue, and even potential injury risk (Pontillo et al., 2020; Watkins et al., 2017).

Research has demonstrated differences in force*time curve characteristics between skilled and unskilled jumpers as well as strong and weak jumpers with stronger and more skilled jumpers generating more force over shorter periods of time (Cormie et al., 2010b; Garhammer & Gregor, 1992). The stronger, more skilled jumpers are able to accelerate their body mass faster and ultimately jump higher than their lesser skilled counterparts.

Countermovement Vertical Jump

The CMVJ can be divided into five phases: unweighting, braking, propulsion, flight, and landing (figure 8.2). The countermovement encompasses the unweighting and braking phases, where the athlete flexes the knees and hips, and dorsiflexes the ankles, lowering the body's center of mass and eccentrically loading the muscles that will propel the body upward. The propulsive phase involves the rapid concentric hip and knee extension and ankle plantar flexion. It begins at the end of the braking phase (the end of the countermovement) and ends when the feet leave the ground (takeoff). The flight phase is when the body is in the air and away from the support surface. Lastly, the landing phase begins when the feet return to the support surface and encompasses the movement and forces necessary for a coordinated landing.

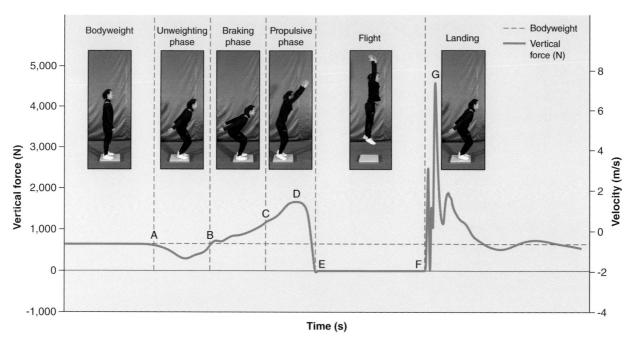

Figure 8.2   Phases of the countermovement vertical jump.

Force*Time Graphs of Various Human Movement Patterns

Identify on the graphs in figures 8.3, 8.4, and 8.5, the points at which each listed event occurs.

Initial foot contact

Peak impact (braking) force

Time to peak impact force

Midstance or foot flat

Peak propulsive force

Time to peak propulsive force

Toe-off

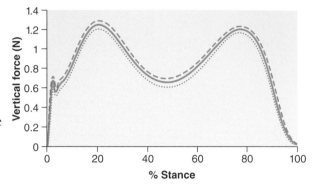

Figure 8.3 Force*time graph of a step during a walking gait.

Initial foot contact

Peak impact force

Time to peak impact force

Peak propulsive force

Time to peak propulsive force

Toe-off

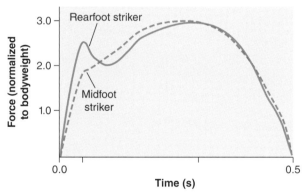

Figure 8.4 Force*time graph of a step during a running gait.

Beginning of the countermovement (unweighting phase)

Maximum downward movement velocity of jumper's center of mass

End of unweighting phase and beginning of braking phase

End of braking phase and beginning of propulsive phase

Peak force

Maximum upward movement velocity of jumper's center of mass

Takeoff

The highest vertical displacement of the jumper's center of mass

End of flight phase and beginning of landing phase

Peak landing impact force

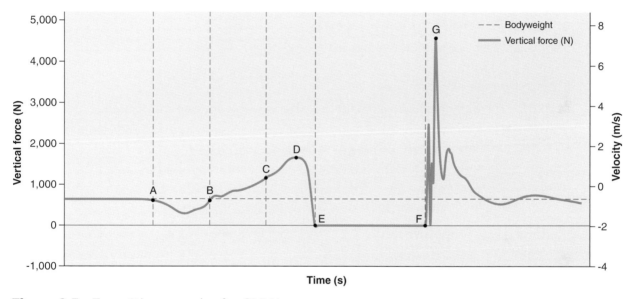

Figure 8.5   Force*time graph of a CMVJ.

Measuring Ground Reaction Force during CMVJ

Equipment

- Force platform and associated computer software

An Excel data file and an associated video file are provided in HK*Propel* for use with this lab.

WWW

Step 1: Ensure force platform and associated computer software are functioning properly. Set the sampling rate at 1,000 Hz or similarly divisible sample rate.

Step 2: Zero the platform.

Step 3: Choose a student volunteer to stand quietly on the platform with hands on hips.

Step 4: Begin data sampling.

Step 5: Have the participant stand as still as possible for one full second.

Step 6: Have the participant execute a CMVJ while maintaining hands on hips and landing carefully back on the force platform.

Step 7: Have the participant stand quietly until data sampling has ended.

Step 8: Export the data file to Microsoft Excel and distribute a copy of the Excel file to all students for use in completing the lab report.

Force*Time Data Analysis in Excel

Equipment

- CMVJ force data file
- Individual laboratory report

> While it is suggested to have each student build their own Excel file for processing force*time data, an Excel file with a completed template is provided in HK*Propel* for use with this lab.
> WWW

Step 1: Open the Microsoft Excel spreadsheet template associated with this lab as well as the CMVJ force data file from laboratory activity 8.1.

Step 2: If laboratory activity 8.1 was not completed, use the CMVJ force data file provided with this manual.

Step 3: Copy and paste the time and force data from the CMVJ data file into columns A and B.

Step 4: Enter the force plate sampling rate into cell K1. Sampling rate for the provided data file is 1,000 Hz.

Step 5: Enter the equations from table 8.1 into the corresponding variable's column in the spreadsheet.

Step 6: Enter the equations from table 8.2 into the corresponding variable's cell in the spreadsheet in order to determine the specific jump phases.

Step 7: Once the data have been completed and the spreadsheet is functioning properly, graph the force*time data. Select columns A and B, click the Insert tab, and select Scatter with Smooth Lines from the chart options. Be sure to include a title for the graph as well as axis titles and a legend. Ensure the chart is selected by clicking on it. Once you have selected it, click the Design tab and select Add chart elements. Select Chart Title, Axis Titles, and Legend. Title the chart *CMVJ Force*time*. Label the *y*-axis *Force (N)*. Label the *x*-axis *Time (s)*.

Step 8: Add the following points of interest to the chart: start of unweighting phase, end of unweighting phase, end of braking phase, peak force, takeoff, peak displacement, and landing.

Step 9: Repeat the following procedures for all listed variables.

Step 10: Click on either the *x*- or *y*-axis of the chart, then right-click and choose Select Data from the menu.

Step 11: From the Select Data Source window, click the Add option. In the Edit Series window, type the name of the point of interest you want to add to the chart. For example, type *End of unweighting* as the name for the end of the unweighting phase.

Step 12: Place the cursor in the Series X values box and click the cell that corresponds to the time of this event. For the end of unweighting, click cell K22. Then place the cursor in the Series Y values box and click the cell that corresponds to the force value at this event. For the end of unweighting, click cell K23. Once this is done, click the OK button.

Step 13: Repeat these steps for all listed variables.

Step 14: To ensure these points are clearly delineated on the chart, right-click on the chart and select Change Chart Type. From the list of chart types on the left, select Combo. Then select the chart type for each data series included on the chart.

Step 15: Select Scatter with Smooth Lines for the force data series. For all points of interest, select Scatter. Ensure the secondary axis box for each data series is unchecked. Click OK. Each point of interest should appear on the chart as a different color than the force*time data.

Table 8.1 Equations for Calculating Kinematic Data in Excel

Variable or cell name	Equation for calculation	Excel formula	Formula location
Net force (N)	=Force – body weight	=B2-$K$6	Cell C2
Acceleration (m/s/s)	=Net force/mass	=C3/$K$7	Cell D3
Velocity (m/s)*	=IF(time point is > integration start time, SUM(velocity from above + (acceleration of row below*time point)),"0.00")	=IF(A3>$K$13,SUM(E2 +(D3*$K$3)),"0.00")	Cell E3
Displacement (m)*	= displacement from previous cell + (velocity of current row*(1/sample frequency))	=F2+(E3*(1/$K$2))	Cell F3

Based on Chavda et al. (2018).

Table 8.2 Equations for Processing CMVJ Data in Excel

Variable or cell name	Equation for calculation	Excel formula
Time point	=1/sample frequency	=1/$K$2
Baseline end	=Baseline start + sample frequency	=K4+$K$2
Body weight (N)	=AVERAGE(INDEX (force array, baseline start):INDEX (force array, baseline end)	=AVERAGE(INDEX(B:B,K4):IN DEX(B:B,K5))
Mass (kg)	=body weight/gravity	=$K$6/9.81
BW – 5 SD value (N)	=body weight – (5 * STDEV.P(INDEX (force array, baseline start):INDEX(force array, baseline end)))	=K6-(5*STDEV.P(INDEX(B:B,K 4):INDEX(B:B,K5)))
BW – 5 SD row	=MATCH(BW – 5 SD value, force array, –1)	=MATCH(K9,B:B,-1)
BW –5 SD time (s)	=INDEX(time array, start row)	=INDEX(A:A,K10)
Integration start time (s)	=BW – 5 SD time (s) – 0.03	=K11-0.03
Integration start row	=MATCH(integration start time, time array, 1)	=MATCH(K13,A:A,1)
Integration start value (N)	=INDEX(net force array, integration start row)	=INDEX(B:B,K14)
Peak force row	=MATCH(MAX(INDEX (force array, first force cell):INDEX(force array, take off row cell)), force array, 0)	=MATCH(MAX(INDEX(B:B,B2): INDEX(B:B,K33)),B:B,0)
Peak force time (s)	=INDEX(time array, peak force row)	=INDEX(A:A,K17)
Peak force value (N)	=INDEX(force array, peak force row)	=INDEX(B:B,K17)
End of unweighting row	=MATCH(MIN(INDEX (velocity array,1): INDEX(velocity array, peak force row)),INDEX (velocity array,1): INDEX(velocity array, peak force row),0)	=MATCH(MIN(INDEX(E:E,1):I NDEX(E:E,K17)),INDEX(E:E,1): INDEX(E:E,K17),0)

Variable or cell name	Equation for calculation	Excel formula
End of unweighting time (s)	=INDEX(time array, end of unweighting row)	=INDEX(A:A,K21)
End of unweighting value (N)	=INDEX(force array, end of unweighting row)	=INDEX(B:B,K21)
End of braking row	=MATCH(0.01,INDEX (velocity array,1): INDEX(velocity array, peak force row),1)	=MATCH(0.01,INDEX(E:E,1):INDEX(E:E,K17),1)
End of braking time (s)	=INDEX(time array, end of braking row)	=INDEX(A:A,K25)
End of braking value (N)	=INDEX(force array, end of braking row)	=INDEX(B:B,K25)
Peak displacement row	=MATCH(MAX (displacement array), displacement array,0)	=MATCH(MAX(F:F),F:F,0)
Peak displacement time (s)	=INDEX(time array, peak displacement row)	=INDEX(A:A,K29)
Peak displacement value (N)	=INDEX(force array, peak displacement row)	=INDEX(B:B,K29)
Takeoff row	=MATCH(10,force array, –1)	=MATCH(10,B:B,-1)
Takeoff time (s)	=INDEX(time array, take off row)	=INDEX(A:A,K33)
Time off value (N)	=INDEX(force array, take off row)	=INDEX(B:B,K33)
Landing row	=MATCH(10,INDEX (force array, peak displacement row): INDEX(force array, (MATCH(MAX(force array)),force array,0))),1) + peak displacement row	=MATCH(10,INDEX(B:B,K29):INDEX(B:B,(MATCH(MAX(B:B), B:B,0))),1)+K29
Landing time (s)	=INDEX(time array, landing row)	=INDEX(A:A,K37)
Landing value (N)	=INDEX(time array, landing row)	=INDEX(B:B,K37)

Based on Chavda et al. (2018).

Laboratory 8 Question Set

Include the CMVJ force*time graph created in Excel as part of your lab report submission. Consider the quiet stance at the beginning of the CMVJ data collection.

1. List the external forces acting on the participant during this time.
2. What can be said about the sum of the total forces acting on the participant while standing still?
3. How would these forces differ for someone with a different mass?
4. Describe how the vertical force changes during the countermovement (unweighting and braking phases) of the jump.

Consider the landing phase of the jump.

1. Why was the peak force experienced during landing so large?
2. Where does this extra force come from?
3. How could the participant decrease the peak force experienced during landing?

Linear Kinetics: Force Variables Influencing Vertical Jump Performance

Objectives

- Examine the force variables affecting vertical jump performance.
- Explain how different jump strategies (fast vs. slow) affect the selected force variables and jump performance.

impulse—The product of a force (N) and the time (s) over which the force is applied. The impulse applied to an object is the cause of and equal to the object's change in momentum.

rate of force development (RFD)—The speed at which the contractile elements of muscle can develop force (Aagaard et al., 2002).

Recall from the previous laboratories that kinetics is the study of the forces that cause or resist motion. Forces can be classified as internal or external, and the external forces that act on a body cause motion. One example of an external force is the ground reaction force that propels the body during walking, running, and jumping. During the countermovement vertical jump (CMVJ), as the body applies force to the ground, the vertical ground reaction force acts on the body to propel it upward and away from the support surface.

The CMVJ is important in sports where gaining vertical jump height can provide an advantage. Examples include jumping to head a corner kick in soccer, blocking a kick in American football, and grabbing a rebound over an opponent in basketball. The goal is to produce force in such a manner that the vertical ground reaction force accelerates the body's center of mass to achieve the highest (or fastest) possible vertical displacement, followed by a coordinated, feet-first landing. Many variables contribute to CMVJ performance. Kinetic variables of impor-

tance include eccentric rate of force development and net concentric impulse (Kirby et al., 2011; Laffaye & Wagner, 2013).

RFD is an important factor in athletic performance in many sporting activities, including sprinting, throwing, and jumping. It is a measure of how fast an athlete can develop muscular force. The application of force (i.e., acceleration) at key time points during sporting activities results in superior performance. For most sporting activities, early force application (i.e., during the initial 50-300 ms) is critical.

Eccentric RFD is calculated as the force developed over the time interval of interest divided by the time interval. The beginning of eccentric RFD calculation corresponds to the end of the unweighting phase of the jump. The end of eccentric RFD calculation corresponds to the end of the braking phase of the jump. Graphically, eccentric RFD is the average slope of the force*time curve during the braking phase of the countermovement. The more vertical the slope, the greater the RFD (see figure 9.1).

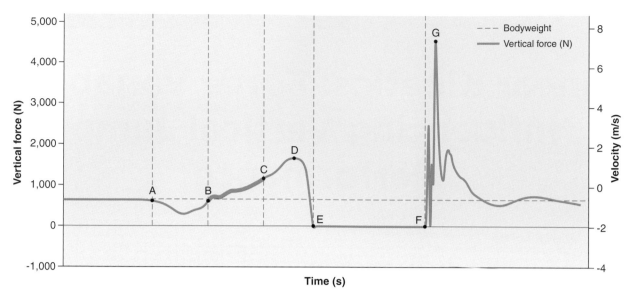

Figure 9.1 Eccentric RFD indicated on a countermovement vertical jump (CMVJ) force*time graph.

Momentum can be thought of as an object's quantity of motion. Linear momentum is the product of an object's mass and its velocity.

$$M = mv$$

$$M = \text{momentum}$$

$$m = \text{mass of the object (kg)}$$

$$v = \text{velocity of the object (m/s)}$$

$$\text{Impulse} = Ft$$

$$F = \text{force (N)}$$

$$t = \text{time (s)}$$

The relationship between impulse and momentum is derived from Newton's second law of motion and is expressed as the impulse–momentum relationship.

$$F = ma$$

$$F = m((v_2 - v_1)/t)$$

$$Ft = (mv_2 - mv_1)$$

$$Ft = \Delta M$$

Jump height has a perfect correlation with impulse (Winter, 2005). In other words, the velocity of the body's movement (i.e., momentum) at CMVJ takeoff is the direct result of the impulse produced by the athlete.

Net concentric impulse is calculated as the product of the net force produced by the athlete and the time over which that net force is produced. The calculation begins at the end of the braking phase (beginning of the propulsive phase) and ends when concentric force passes below body weight. Graphically, it is represented as the area between the force*time curve but above body weight (see figure 9.2).

The use of force platforms to assess CMVJ performance can reveal an athlete's ability in regard to these kinetic variables. Further, frequent and consistent monitoring of these variables can provide insight into athlete readiness and fatigue, as well as inform exercise training decisions.

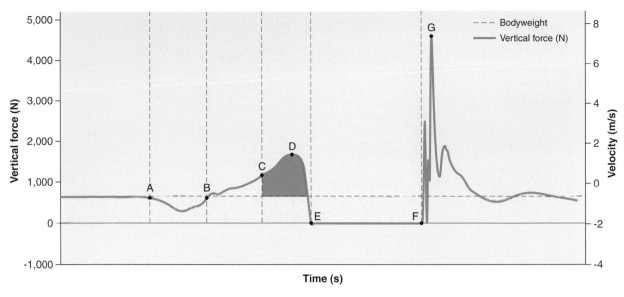

Figure 9.2   Net concentric impulse represented on a CMVJ force*time graph.

Calculating Eccentric RFD and Net Concentric Impulse in Excel

Equipment

- Completed Microsoft Excel spreadsheet template from chapter 8
- Individual laboratory report

Step 1:   Open the completed Microsoft Excel spreadsheet template from chapter 8.

Step 2:   Enter the impulse equation from the individual laboratory report into the Impulse column (column G) in the spreadsheet.

Step 3:   Enter the equations for eccentric RFD, net concentric impulse, and jump height from the individual laboratory report into the corresponding cell for each variable in the spreadsheet.

Measuring Ground Reaction Force During Different CMVJ Techniques

Equipment

- Force platform and associated computer software
- CMVJ force data files
- Microsoft Excel and completed Excel template file from chapter 8

> Excel data files (jump executed quickly vs. jump executed slowly) are provided in HK*Propel* for use with this lab.
>
> www

Step 1: Ensure force platform and associated computer software are functioning properly. Set sampling rate at 1,000 Hz or similarly divisible sample rate.

Step 2: Zero the platform.

Step 3: Have a participant stand quietly on the platform with hands on hips.

Step 4: Begin data sampling.

Step 5: Have the participant stand as still as possible for 1 full second.

Step 6: Have the participant execute a CMVJ as quickly as possible while maintaining hands on hips and landing carefully back on the force platform.

Step 7: Have the participant stand quietly until data sampling has ended.

Step 8: Save the data file.

Step 9: Repeat the CMVJ data collection procedures listed previously, but this time, have the participant execute the CMVJ by moving more slowly through the eccentric and concentric phases of the jump.

Step 10: Export both CMVJ data files to Microsoft Excel and distribute copies of the files to all students for use in completing the lab report.

Examining Force Variables From Different CMVJ Techniques

Equipment

- Completed Microsoft Excel spreadsheet template from laboratory activity 9.1
- CMVJ data files
- Microsoft Excel
- Laboratory report

Step 1: Open the completed Microsoft Excel spreadsheet template from laboratory activity 9.1. Insert two new tabs and copy and paste the data template into those new tabs. Rename one tab *Fast CMVJ* and the other tab *Slow CMVJ*.

Step 2: Enter the force plate sampling rate into cell K1 for both new tabs. Sampling rate for the provided data file is 1,000 Hz.

Step 3: Replace the force*time data from laboratory activity 9.1 with the force*time data collected during laboratory activity 9.2.

Step 4: Place the fast jump data into the Fast CMVJ tab and the slow jump data into the Slow CMVJ tab. If laboratory activity 9.2 was not completed, use the CMVJ force data files provided for use with this lab.

Step 5: Graph the force*time data for both jumps. Select columns A and B, click the Insert tab, and select Scatter with Smooth Lines from the chart options.

Step 6: Include a title for the graph as well as axis titles and a legend. Ensure the chart is selected by clicking on it. Once it is selected, click the Design tab and select Add chart elements. Select Chart Title, Axis Titles, and Legend. Label the chart title *CMVJ Force*time*. Label the *y*-axis *Force (N)*. Label the *x*-axis *Time (s)*.

Step 7: Add the following points of interest to the chart: start of unweighting phase, end of unweighting phase, end of braking phase, peak force, takeoff, peak displacement, and landing. To do this, repeat the following procedures for all listed variables. Click on either the *x*- or *y*- axis of the chart, then right click and choose Select Data from the menu. Click Add in the Select Data Source window. In the Edit Series window, type the name of the point of interest you want to add to the chart. For example, type *End of Unweighting* as the name for the end of the unweighting phase.

Step 8: Place the cursor in the Series X values box and click the cell that corresponds to the time of this event. For the end of unweighting, click cell K22.

Step 9: Place the cursor in the Series Y values box and click the cell that corresponds to the force value at this event. For the end of unweighting, click cell K23. Once this is done, click the OK button. Repeat these steps for all listed variables.

Step 10: To ensure these points are clearly delineated on the chart, right click on the chart and select Change Chart Type. From the list of chart types on the left, select Combo. Then, select the chart type for each data series included on the chart. Select Scatter with Smooth Lines for the force data series. For all points of interest, select Scatter. Ensure the secondary axis box for each data series is unchecked. Click OK. Each point of interest should appear on the chart as a different color than the force*time data.

Step 11: Use these completed templates and the associated graphs to complete the laboratory report.

INDIVIDUAL LABORATORY REPORT

Variable or cell name	Equation for calculation	Excel formula	Formula location
Impulse (Ns)	= (Average of (current row and previous row of net force)) * (1 / sample frequency)	=(AVERAGE(C2:C3))*(1/$K$1)	Cell G3

Variable or cell name	Equation for calculation	Excel formula
Eccentric RFD	=((INDEX (force array, end of unweighting row)) − (INDEX (force array, end of braking row)))/ (end of unweighting time − end of braking time)	=((INDEX(B:B,$K$25))-(INDEX(B:B,$K$21)))/($K$26-$K$22)
Net concentric impulse	=SUM(INDEX(impulse array, end of braking row):INDEX(impulse array, takeoff row 5 SD))	=SUM(INDEX(G:G,$K$25):INDEX(G:G,$K$42))
Jump height	=SUM(INDEX(velocity array, takeoff row)^2)/(2*9.81)	=SUM(INDEX(E:E,$K$33)^2)/(2*9.81)

Insert the eccentric RFD, net concentric impulse, and jump height variables calculated in laboratory activity 9.1.

Eccentric RFD _____

Net concentric impulse _____

Jump height _____

From J. Garner, C. Allen, H. Chander, and A. Knight, *Applied Biomechanics Laboratory Manual.* (Champaign, IL: Human Kinetics, 2023).

LABORATORY ACTIVITY 9.3

INDIVIDUAL LABORATORY REPORT

Insert the eccentric RFD, net concentric impulse, and jump height variables calculated in laboratory activity 9.3 for both the Fast CMVJ and the Slow CMVJ files.

Fast CMVJ File

Eccentric RFD _____

Net concentric impulse _____

Jump height _____

Slow CMVJ File

Eccentric RFD _____

Net concentric impulse _____

Jump height _____

Copy the graphs of the force*time curves for both the Fast CMVJ and Slow CMVJ files and include them in this report.

Which jump, the fast or slow CMVJ, led to a higher vertical displacement? Why? In your response, include discussion of both eccentric RFD and net concentric impulse.

How does eccentric RFD differ between the two jumps?

How does net concentric impulse differ between the two jumps?

From J. Garner, C. Allen, H. Chander, and A. Knight, *Applied Biomechanics Laboratory Manual.* (Champaign, IL: Human Kinetics, 2023).

Angular Kinetics and Levers

Objectives

- Understand the principles of angular kinetics.
- Learn the different types of levers found in the body.
- Calculate torque production.

DEFINITIONS

braking torque—A torque that will decrease the velocity of a rotating segment.

lever—A rigid body that is used with an axis to multiply the force or speed applied to another body.

lever arm (l)—The distance from the axis of rotation to the point of force application.

moment arm (⊥d)—The perpendicular distance from the force vector to the axis of rotation.

propulsive torque—A torque that will increase the velocity of a rotating segment.

torque or moment of force (T or M)—The turning effect of a force. Torque, or moment, is the product of force (F) and moment arm (⊥d), or the product of the perpendicular component of force (⊥F) and the lever arm (l).

$$T = F \times \perp d, \text{ or } T = \perp F \times l$$

This lab introduces the principles of angular kinetics and their application to the various fields of sport performance, ergonomics, and injury rehabilitation, primarily through the use of levers. In order for an object or body segment to rotate, a force that causes rotation must be applied. Angular kinetics deals with the rotatory effects of forces. A torque, or moment of force, is the turning effect of a force. The ability of a force to cause rotation is determined by the magnitude of the force, the perpendicular component of the force, and the length of the moment arm. A good example is opening a door. In order to cause a door to rotate and open, you must apply a force to the door. The farther away from the door you apply the force, and the greater the perpendicular component of the force, the easier it is to open the door. If you apply the force near the hinges of the door, you have to apply a large amount of force due to the short length of the moment arm.

APPLICATION TO HUMAN MOVEMENT

When we actively move our limbs, our muscles contract and apply a force to our bones, and if the torque produced by this force is greater than the torque produced by the resistance, it causes our bones to rotate, and angular motion will occur. This turning effect that our muscular forces have on our bony segments is a torque or moment of force. Since the human body is a series of connected semirigid links, these articulations can be modeled after simple machines called levers. Each type of simple machine must serve one or more of the following functions: (1) balance two or more forces, (2) change the direction of the applied force, (3) favor force production, or (4) favor speed and range of motion. Later, we will examine how different levers in the body can serve each of these functions.

Each lever consists of five primary components. These include (1) the axis of rotation (the joint that is rotating), (2) the applied force (in the body, this is the muscular force applied to the bony segment), (3) the resistance force (the load that has to be overcome), (4) the force moment arm, and (5) the resistance moment arm. The force moment arm can be defined as the perpendicular distance from the force vector of the muscle that is contracting to the axis of rotation, and the resistance moment arm is the perpendicular distance from the force vector of the resistance to the axis of rotation.

Levers can be classified into three different groups. While there are five components to each lever, only three of these components are used to classify them. These components are the force (F), the axis (A), and the resistance (R). In a first-class lever, the axis is always between the force and the resistance (FAR or RAF). In a second-class lever, the resistance is always between the force and the axis (FRA or ARF). In a third-class lever, the force is always between the axis and the resistance (AFR or RFA). The function of each lever will be discussed in more detail.

First-Class Lever

In a first-class lever, the axis is always between the force and the resistance (FAR or RAF). This is the most versatile lever because depending on the position of the axis, it can potentially serve all four of the functions of a simple machine (figure 10.1).

- **Balance two forces:** Since both the force and the resistance are the same distance from the axis, and each has the same moment arm,

the amount of force required to balance the resistance is equal to the magnitude of the resistance.

- **Change the effective direction of the applied force:** In previous example, if the force applied is greater than the resistance, then the force end of the lever will move down, and the resistance end will move up.

- **Favor speed and range of motion:** In figure 10.2, the axis is closer to the force than the resistance. This means that the resistance end of the lever will move a greater distance than the force end of the lever, in the same time period. A greater amount of distance covered in the same time period equals a greater amount of speed. The disadvantage of this arrangement is that it takes a large amount of force to move the resistance, since the resistance moment arm is much greater than the force moment arm.

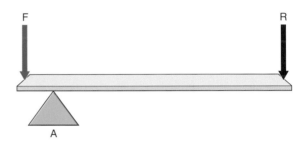

Figure 10.2 A first class lever that is designed to favor speed and range of motion.

- **Favor force production:** In figure 10.3, the axis is now much closer to the resistance. This means the force moment arm is much longer than the resistance moment arm, and it does not take as much force to move the resistance.

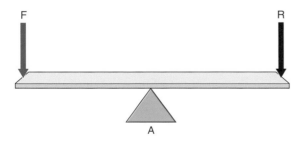

Figure 10.1 A first class lever that is designed to balance two forces.

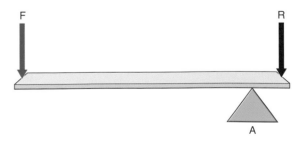

Figure 10.3 A first class lever that is designed to favor force production.

• **Example within the body:** Neck extension. The arrangement shown in figure 10.4 is designed to balance two forces—in this case, the force from the neck extensors on the posterior side of the head and neck, and the resistance provided by the weight of the skull. This arrangement is beneficial for us to keep our head level.

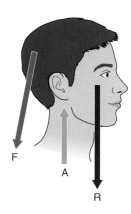

Figure 10.4 F is supplied by the neck extensors. A is at the spine or skull articulation. R is supplied by the weight of the head, considered to act at the R center of gravity of the skull.

Second-Class Lever

In a second-class lever, the resistance is always between the axis of rotation and the force (ARF or FRA). Due to this arrangement, the force moment arm will always be longer than the resistance moment arm. This arrangement will favor force production, because a smaller force will be required to move a larger load due to the longer force moment arm. While this configuration is the most efficient for force production, it is not a common arrangement in the body. The arrangement of a second class lever can be seen in figure 10.5.

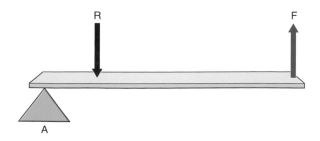

Figure 10.5 The arrangement of the components in a second class lever.

• **Example within the body:** Toe raise. This arrangement (figure 10.6) favors force production by the gastrocnemius–soleus–Achilles tendon complex (triceps surae).

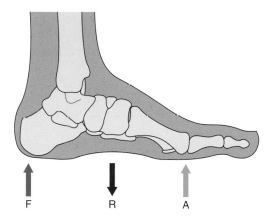

Figure 10.6 A is at the metatarsal phalange joint; R is supplied by the weight of the person acting through the center of gravity; and F is supplied by the gastrocnemius and soleus muscles through the attachment of the Achilles tendon.

Third-Class Lever

In this class of lever, the force is always between the axis and the resistance. This means the resistance moment arm is always longer than the force moment arm, and therefore, it will take a larger amount of force to move the resistance. The benefit of this arrangement is that it will favor speed and range of motion. If you look at figure 10.7, it is clear that while the force end of the lever will only move a small distance, the resistance end of the lever will move a much greater distance in the same time period. Therefore, the resistance end of the lever is moving faster than the force end of the lever.

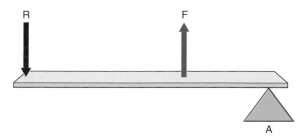

Figure 10.7 The arrangement of the components of a third class lever.

The third-class lever is the most common type of lever in the human body. Most of our muscles attach close to the joint that they cross, meaning the joint serves as the axis, the force is located near the axis, and the resistance is located at the end of the lever. Therefore, the human body is designed for speed and range of motion, but this arrangement does require the development of a large amount of force to overcome the resistance. An example of a third class lever can be seen in figure 10.8. We will calculate these numbers in the next section.

- **Example within the body:** Dumbbell curl.

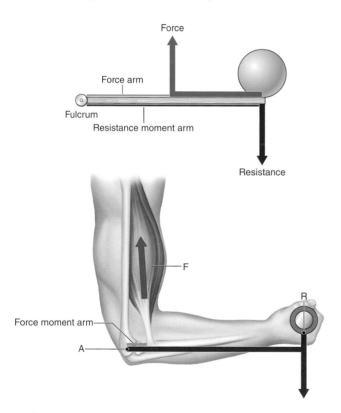

Figure 10.8 A is at the humeroulnar joint; F is supplied by muscular force (insertion of the elbow flexors); and R is supplied by the load in the hand.

CALCULATING TORQUE OR MOMENT OF FORCE

When you calculate the torque or moment of force produced by a muscle, you have to multiply the force produced by the muscle by the moment arm for the muscle. To calculate the torque or moment produced by the resistance, you have to multiply the amount of force produced by the resistance by the moment arm for the resistance. In human movement, the resistance moment arm is almost always longer than the force moment arm (because we are primarily composed of class three levers), so our muscles must produce a large amount of force to overcome the torque produced by the resistance. An example of this is the elbow flexion, and more specifically, the upward phase of a dumbbell curl. If we know the magnitude of the resistance, the length of the resistance moment arm, and the length of the force moment arm, then we can calculate how much force the elbow flexors must produce to balance the torque produced by the dumbbell and how much force the elbow flexors must produce to overcome the torque produced by the resistance and cause the elbow to move into flexion, which would lift the dumbbell up toward the shoulder. In this example and other examples, we will use the weight of a dumbbell or cuff weight in pounds, but this needs to be converted into newtons (N). One pound is equal to 4.45 N.

Dumbbell Curl

Equipment

- 20 lb (89 N) dumbbell

Data Needed to Complete Activity

Axis of rotation: Humeroulnar joint

Applied force: Elbow flexors

Resistance: Dumbbell

Force moment arm ($\perp d$): Perpendicular distance from the attachment of the elbow flexors (just distal to the elbow) to the joint center of the elbow.

Resistance moment arm ($\perp d$): Perpendicular distance from the dumbbell to the elbow joint center (think about the distance from a dumbbell in your hand to the elbow).

Dumbbell: 20 lb × 4.45 N/lb = 89 N

Resistance moment arm ($\perp d$ dumbbell): 0.38 m

Applied force (muscular force) from the elbow flexors: To be determined

Force moment arm ($\perp d$ elbow flexors): 0.048 m

We are going to solve for how much force the elbow flexors must produce to balance the torque provided by the dumbbell, and how much force the elbow flexors must produce to overcome the resistance of the dumbbell. There is a three-step process to follow, which is outlined shortly. You can record your findings in the table.

Amount of muscular force	Length of moment arm for the muscular force	Muscular torque	Amount of resistance	Length of moment arm for the resistance	Torque produced by the resistance
	0.048 m		89 N	0.38 m	

Step 1: Solve for the torque produced by the dumbbell.

$$T_{dumbbell} = F_{dumbbell} \times \perp d_{dumbbell}$$

$$T = 89 \text{ N} \times 0.38 \ m$$

$$T = 33.82 \text{ N m}$$

The dumbbell produces 33.82 N m of torque. This torque will cause the elbow to move into extension.

Step 2: Solve for the force produced by the elbow flexors.

The elbow flexors must produce 33.82 N m of torque to balance the torque produced by the dumbbell and keep the forearm in a static position. The moment arm for the elbow flexors is 0.048 m.

$$F_{elbow\ flexors} \times \perp d_{elbow\ flexors} = 33.82\ N\ m$$

$$F_{elbow\ flexors} \times 0.048\ m = 33.82\ N\ m$$

$$F_{elbow\ flexors} = 33.82\ N\ m/0.048\ m$$

$$F_{elbow\ flexors} = 704.58\ N$$

The elbow flexors must produce 704.58 N of force to balance the torque produced by the dumbbell.

Step 3: If the elbow flexors must produce 704.58 N of force to balance the torque produced by the dumbbell, then any amount of force greater than 704.58 N will produce a torque that overcomes the torque produced by the dumbbell. So, the answer is the elbow flexors must produce greater than 704.58 N of force to overcome the resistance provided by the dumbbell and cause the elbow to move into flexion.

We can see in this scenario that if the dumbbell has a weight of 89 N, the elbow flexors must produce greater than 704.58 N of force to overcome the torque produced by this weight. Remember, elbow flexion is an example of a third-class lever, meaning the moment arm for the resistance is much greater than the moment arm for the force. The advantage of this arrangement is that the distal end of the forearm and hand will move a much greater distance in the same time period compared to the proximal end of the forearm where the elbow flexors insert, which favors speed and range of motion, but it does require a large amount of force from the elbow flexors to balance or overcome the torque produced by the elbow flexors.

From a practical standpoint, the preceding example demonstrates that there are two ways to reduce the amount of torque produced by the resistance. You can either reduce the amount of the resistance (choose a lighter weight) or reduce the distance of the resistance from the axis of rotation. For a dumbbell curl, it is not possible to move the dumbbell closer to the elbow, but it is possible to choose a lighter dumbbell. If a therapist or athletic trainer is using a cuff weight as the resistance, then it is possible to move the cuff weight closer to the axis of rotation. For example, if a patient is performing a seated knee extension exercise, the therapist or athletic trainer could move the cuff weight closer to the knee, which would reduce the moment arm of the cuff weight and the amount of torque produced by the cuff weight.

Identifying Levers in the Body

Equipment

- Individual laboratory report
- Another person to help visualize the levers

For the following joint actions, determine if it should be classified as a first-class, second-class, or third-class lever. Identify the axis of rotation, the applied muscular force, the resistance, the force moment arm, and the resistance moment arm. Record your findings in the appropriate column in the table in the individual laboratory report. If there is no external resistance, you can consider the resistance to be the weight of the segment, such as the forearm or hand or the shank or foot.

1. Knee extension
   a. Type of lever: _____
   b. Axis of rotation: _____
   c. Applied muscular force: _____
   d. Resistance: _____
   e. Force moment arm: _____
   f. Resistance moment arm: _____

2. Hip flexion
   a. Type of lever: _____
   b. Axis of rotation: _____
   c. Applied muscular force: _____
   d. Resistance: _____
   e. Force moment arm: _____
   f. Resistance moment arm: _____

3. Shoulder abduction
   a. Type of lever: _____
   b. Axis of rotation: _____
   c. Applied muscular force: _____
   d. Resistance: _____
   e. Force moment arm: _____
   f. Resistance moment arm: _____

4. Elbow extension
   a. Type of lever: _____
   b. Axis of rotation: _____
   c. Applied muscular force: _____
   d. Resistance: _____
   e. Force moment arm: _____
   f. Resistance moment arm: _____

5. Ankle dorsiflexion
    a. Type of lever: _____
    b. Axis of rotation: _____
    c. Applied muscular force: _____
    d. Resistance: _____
    e. Force moment arm: _____
    f. Resistance moment arm: _____

Seated Knee Extension Exercise With a Cuff Weight

Equipment

- 15 lb (66.75 N) cuff weight
- Individual laboratory report

Data Needed to Complete Activity

Cuff weight: 15 lb (remember 1 lb equals 4.45 N)

Resistance moment arm: 0.48 m

Applied force: To be determined

Force moment arm: 0.052 m

How much force must the quadriceps produce to balance the torque provided by the cuff weight? How much force must the quadriceps produce to overcome the resistance of the cuff weight?

Step 1:   Solve for the torque produced by the cuff weight.

a. _____

b. _____

c. _____

Step 2:   Solve for the force produced by the quadriceps.

a. _____

b. _____

c. _____

d. _____

e. _____

f. _____

g. The quadriceps must produce _____ N of force to balance the torque produced by the resistance.

Step 3:   How much force must the quadriceps produce to overcome the torque produced by the cuff weight?

LABORATORY 10.3 ACTIVITY

INDIVIDUAL LABORATORY REPORT

For the following joint actions, determine what type of lever it would be classified as. Identify the axis of rotation, the applied muscular force, the resistance, the force moment arm, and the resistance moment arm.

1. Knee flexion
   a. Type of lever:
   b. Axis of rotation:
   c. Applied muscular force:
   d. Resistance:
   e. Force moment arm:
   f. Resistance moment arm:

2. Hip extension
   a. Type of lever:
   b. Axis of rotation:
   c. Applied muscular force:
   d. Resistance:
   e. Force moment arm:
   f. Resistance moment arm:

3. Shoulder adduction
   a. Type of lever:
   b. Axis of rotation:
   c. Applied muscular force:
   d. Resistance:
   e. Force moment arm:
   f. Resistance moment arm:

4. Hip abduction
   a. Type of lever:
   b. Axis of rotation:
   c. Applied muscular force:
   d. Resistance:
   e. Force moment arm:
   f. Resistance moment arm:

From J. Garner, C. Allen, H. Chander, and A. Knight, *Applied Biomechanics Laboratory Manual.* (Champaign, IL: Human Kinetics, 2023).

5. Ankle plantar flexion

    a. Type of lever:

    b. Axis of rotation:

    c. Applied muscular force:

    d. Resistance:

    e. Force moment arm:

    f. Resistance moment arm:

From J. Garner, C. Allen, H. Chander, and A. Knight, *Applied Biomechanics Laboratory Manual.* (Champaign, IL: Human Kinetics, 2023).

Prone Knee Flexion Exercise With a Cuff Weight

Equipment

- 25 lb (111.25 N) cuff weight
- Individual laboratory report

Data Needed to Complete Activity

Cuff weight: 25 lb (111.25 N)

Resistance moment arm: 0.45 m

Applied force: To be determined

Force moment arm: 0.054 m

How much force must the hamstrings produce to balance the torque provided by the cuff weight? How much force must the hamstrings produce to overcome the resistance of the cuff weight?

Step 1: Solve for the torque produced by the cuff weight.

    a.

    b.

    c.

Step 2: Solve for the force produced by the hamstrings.

    a.

    b.

    c.

    d.

    e.

    f. The quadriceps must produce _____ N of force to balance the torque produced by the resistance.

Step 3: How much force must the hamstrings produce to overcome the torque produced by the cuff weight?

INDIVIDUAL LABORATORY REPORT

1. Cervical or neck flexion
   a. Type of lever:
   b. Axis of rotation:
   c. Applied muscular force:
   d. Resistance:
   e. Force moment arm:
   f. Resistance moment arm:

2. Wrist extension
   a. Type of lever:
   b. Axis of rotation:
   c. Applied muscular force:
   d. Resistance:
   e. Force moment arm:
   f. Resistance moment arm:

3. Shoulder flexion
   a. Type of lever:
   b. Axis of rotation:
   c. Applied muscular force:
   d. Resistance:
   e. Force moment arm:
   f. Resistance moment arm:

4. Elbow adduction
   a. Type of lever:
   b. Axis of rotation:
   c. Applied muscular force:
   d. Resistance:
   e. Force moment arm:
   f. Resistance moment arm:

5. Ankle dorsiflexion (tibialis anterior)
   a. Type of lever:
   b. Axis of rotation:
   c. Applied muscular force:
   d. Resistance:
   e. Force moment arm:
   f. Resistance moment arm:

From J. Garner, C. Allen, H. Chander, and A. Knight, *Applied Biomechanics Laboratory Manual.* (Champaign, IL: Human Kinetics, 2023).

Work, Power, and Energy

Objectives

- Understand the principles of work, power, and energy.
- Apply the principles of work, power, and energy to human movement.
- Understand mechanical energy in its two primary forms: kinetic energy and potential energy.
- Analyze the transformation of mechanical energy during movement.

DEFINITIONS

energy—The state of matter that makes things change or has the potential to make things change.

gravitational potential energy—The potential energy (PE) that a body has due to its position.

$$PE = m \times a_g \times h$$
(a_g = acceleration due to gravity)

kinetic energy—The energy that a body has due to its motion, or more simply, the energy due to motion. An object must be moving to possess kinetic energy (must have a velocity). A person or object must have a linear velocity or angular velocity in order to have kinetic energy. The velocity variable is a squared value, so it does have more influence on kinetic energy than mass or moment of inertia.

- Equation for linear kinetic energy—

$$E_{LK} = \frac{1}{2}m \times v^2$$

- Equation for angular (rotational) kinetic energy—

$$E_{AK} = \frac{1}{2}I \times \omega^2$$

potential energy—The energy a body has that has the potential to change something but is not currently changing anything, or more simply, the energy due to position or deformation.

power—The amount of work done within a certain time period, or the rate at which force is applied.

strain potential energy—The energy a body has due to its deformation. Objects that can return to their original shape after being deformed (lengthened, squashed, twisted) can store energy while they are being deformed.

work—A measure of the amount of force that has been applied over a certain displacement.

Since energy can be neither created nor destroyed, the total energy of a system will remain constant. We are going to primarily deal with linear kinetic energy and gravitational potential energy.

The unit for energy is a joule (J). Energy is a scalar quantity, so it only has a magnitude.

WORK

Work is the process of changing the amount of energy in a system. Work is the product of force and displacement. If a person or object does not undergo displacement, then no work has occurred. Mathematically, work can be represented by the following equation: $W = F \times \Delta p$. For angular movements, work is the product of torque and angular displacement: $W = T \times \Delta \mu$.

A person applies 500 N of force to move an object 15 m. How much work have they done?

$$W = (500 \text{ N})(15 \text{ m}); W = 7,500 \text{ J}$$

The biceps muscle produces 78 Nm of torque to move a dumbbell through an angular displacement of 2.0 rad. How much work has the biceps done?

$$W = (78 \text{ Nm})(2.0 \text{ rad}) = 156 \text{ J}$$

POWER

Power is the time rate of doing work. Power is work divided by time, or force multiplied by velocity in the linear sense, and torque multiplied by angular velocity in the angular sense.

$$P = \frac{W}{\Delta t} = \frac{\Delta E}{\Delta t} = \frac{F \times \Delta p}{\Delta t} = F \times \frac{\Delta p}{\Delta t} = F \times v$$

$$P\frac{W}{\Delta t} = \frac{\Delta E}{\Delta t} = \frac{T \times \Delta\theta}{\Delta t} = T \times \frac{\Delta\theta}{\Delta t} = T \times \omega$$

If a person does 7,500 J of work in 10 s, what is their power output?

$$P = (7,500 \text{ J})/(10 \text{ s}); P = 750 \text{ W}$$

If a person applies 250 N of force to move an object at a velocity of 5 m/s, what is their power output?

$$P = (250 \text{ N})(5 \text{ m/s}) = 1,250 \text{ W}$$

The unit of measurement for power is watts (W).

Previous chapters have examined the cause of motion (force and torque), impulse, momentum, and other concepts related to Newton's laws of motion. These concepts and techniques are very useful to analyze human movement, but there are other techniques and concepts that are very valuable as well. This includes the concepts of work, power, and energy, and how they can be used to further understand and analyze human movement.

CALCULATING ENERGY

Due to the first law of thermodynamics, energy is neither created nor destroyed, but it can change from one form to another. During human movement, there is a transfer of energy from kinetic to potential energy when a person moves up, and a transfer from potential energy to kinetic energy when a person moves down. Total energy will be equal to the sum of kinetic energy plus potential energy.

For the first example, we will examine the potential energy, kinetic energy, total energy, and velocity of a person as they jump off a 10 m high diving platform. This will allow us to isolate what happens to energy and velocity as a person moves down. We will later add the upward component as well by examining the upward and downward phase of a jump. For this first example, we will assume the person has a mass of 55 kg. The person is starting at the top of a 10 m high diving platform (figure 11.1). We will solve for their potential energy, kinetic energy, total energy, and velocity at different points along the dive.

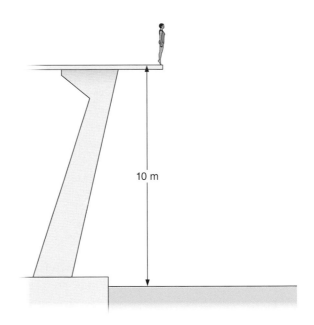

Figure 11.1 A person stands on the top of a 10 m diving platform.

- Potential energy: $PE = m \star a_g \star h$, $PE = (55 \text{ kg})(9.81 \text{ m/s}^2)(10 \text{ m})$. Since energy is a scalar, we do not have to include the negative sign when multiplying by the acceleration due to gravity. *This only holds true when calculating energy.*

$$PE = 5,395.5 \text{ J}$$

- Kinetic energy: $KE = \frac{1}{2} \star m \star v^2 = KE = \frac{1}{2}(55 \text{ kg})(0 \text{ m/s})$, since the person is not moving, his or her velocity is 0 m/s.

$$KE = 0 \text{ J}$$

- Total energy: $TE = KE + PE$; $TE = 0 \text{ J} + 5,395.5 \text{ J}$; $TE = 5,395.5 \text{ J}$. Total energy will remain the same for the entire movement from the top of the diving platform to the water; it will just change from potential energy to kinetic energy as the person moves down.

- Velocity: $v = 0$ m/s (because the person isn't moving).

In figure 11.2, the person is 6 m from the water (4 m from the top of the diving platform).

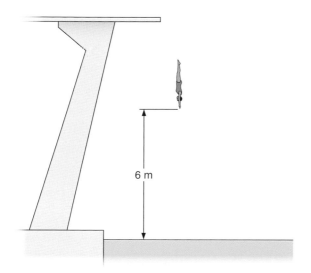

Figure 11.2 A person has dived off a 10 m diving platform and is 6 m above the water.

As the person moves down toward the water, their potential energy will decrease (because their height above the water is decreasing), but their kinetic energy will increase (because velocity is increasing).

- Total energy: TE = 5,395.5 J (remember, this will not change). If you solve correctly for potential energy to start with, this value will remain the same throughout the entire movement.
- Potential energy: PE = m*a_g*h, PE = (55 kg) (9.81 m/s²)(6 m).

$$PE = 3,237.3 \text{ J (potential energy}$$
has decreased because height above
the water has decreased)

- Kinetic energy: Since TE = KE + PE, KE = TE – PE, so KE = 5,395.5 J – 3,237.3 J, KE = 2, 158.2 J.
- Velocity: Since we know kinetic energy, we can use this equation to solve for velocity.
- KE = ½ m*v^2; 2,158.2 J = ½ (55 kg)(v^2); 2,158.2 J = (27.5 kg)(v^2); 2,158.2 J/27.5 kg = v^2;

78.48 $m^2/s^2 = v^2$; $\sqrt{78.48} = v$; $v = -8.86$ m/s. Velocity is negative because the person is moving down towards the water in the negative vertical direction.

In figure 11.3, the person is 3 m from the water (7 m from the top of the diving platform).

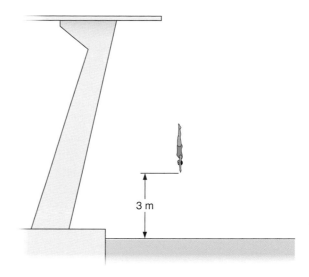

Figure 11.3 A person has dived off a 10 m diving platform and is 3 m above the water.

As the person continues to move down toward the water, his or her potential energy will continue to decrease (because their height above the water is still decreasing), but their kinetic energy will continue to increase (because velocity is still increasing).

- Total energy: TE = 5, 395.5 J (remember, this will not change).
- Potential energy: PE = m*a_g*h, PE = (55 kg) (9.81 m/s^2)(3 m).

$$PE = 1,618.65 \text{ J (potential energy}$$
has continued to decrease)

- Kinetic energy: Since TE = KE + PE, KE = TE – PE, so KE = 5,395.5 J – 1,618.65 J, so KE = 3,776.85 J.
- Velocity: Since we know kinetic energy, we can use this equation to solve for velocity.
- KE = ½ mv^2; 3,776.85 J = ½ (55 kg)(v^2); 3,776.85 J = (27.5 kg)(v^2); 3.776.85 J/27.5 kg = v^2; 137.4 $m^2/s^2 = v^2$; $\sqrt{137.34} = v$; $v = -11.72$ m/s. Velocity is negative because the person is

moving down toward the water in the negative vertical direction.

For the second example, we will examine the potential energy, kinetic energy, total energy, and velocity of a person as they perform a vertical jump. Let's assume the person has a mass of 75 kg. They perform a vertical jump with an initial vertical velocity of 5 m/s. What is their potential energy, kinetic energy, total energy, and velocity at different points along the trajectory of the jump?

When the person takes off, they have an initial velocity, but they are not off the ground yet (or they are just leaving the ground). Therefore, they would have kinetic energy but no potential energy. As they move toward the apex of their jump, they will gain potential energy (because their height is increasing) and lose kinetic energy (because their velocity is decreasing). At the apex of the jump, all of their energy will be in the form of potential energy (remember, vertical velocity at the apex of a jump is 0 m/s, meaning they have no kinetic energy). On the way down, they will lose potential energy and gain kinetic energy (height above the ground is decreasing while velocity is increasing).

At the Beginning of the Jump

- Potential energy: PE = $m \star a_g \star h$, PE = (75 kg) (9.81 m/s²)(0 m); PE = 0 J.
- Kinetic energy: KE = ½ $m \star v^2$; KE = ½ (75 kg)(5 m/s)²; KE = 937.5 J (don't forget to square velocity).
- Total energy: TE = PE + KE; TE = 0 J + 937.5 J; TE = 937.5 J.
- Velocity: 5 m/s.

At the Apex of the Jump

At the apex, we know that all energy will be potential energy, so kinetic energy and velocity are zero. Based on the initial **y** velocity, we can use our equation from projectile motion to solve for the maximum height of the jump, then plug this height into the equation for potential energy to make sure it is equal to (or approximately equal to due to rounding) 937.5 J.

$$h = \frac{v_y^2}{2 * a_g}$$

h = (5 m/s)²/(2)(−9.81 m/s²); h = 25/19.62; h = 1.274 m. This is the maximum height of the jump.

- Potential energy: PE = $m \star a_g \star h$, PE = (75 kg) (9.81 m/s²)(1.274 m); PE = 937.5 J.
- Kinetic energy: KE = ½ $m \star v^2$; KE = ½ (75 kg)(0 m/s)²; KE = 0 J.
- Total energy: TE = KE + PE; TE = 0 J + 937.5 J; TE = 937.5 J.
- Velocity: 0 m/s.

1 m Off the Ground

Let's calculate these variables when the jumper is 1 m off the ground, on his way up.

- Potential energy: PE = $m \star a_g \star h$, PE = (75 kg) (9.81 m/s²)(1 m); PE = 735.75 J.
- Kinetic energy: Since TE = KE + PE, KE = TE − PE, so KE = 937.5 J − 735.75 J, so KE = 201.75 J.
- Velocity: Since we know kinetic energy, we can use this equation to solve for velocity.
- KE = ½ $m \star v^2$; 201.75 J = ½ (75 kg)(v^2); 201.75 J = (37.5 kg)(v^2); 201.75 J/37.5 kg = v^2; m²/s² = v^2; $\sqrt{5.38}$ = v; v = 2.32 m/s. Velocity is positive because the person is moving up toward the apex of their jump in the positive vertical direction.

Calculating Potential Energy, Kinetic Energy, Total Energy, and Velocity

This activity is to be completed in class.

High Diving Platform Problem

A person is jumping off a 5 m high diving platform. Let's assume the person has a mass of 85 kg. What is their potential energy, kinetic energy, total energy, and velocity?

At the Top of the 5 m Diving Platform

$$\text{Potential energy: PE} = m\text{*}a_g\text{*}h$$

$$\text{PE} =$$

$$\text{Kinetic energy: KE} = \tfrac{1}{2}\text{*}m\text{*}v^2$$

$$\text{KE} =$$

$$\text{Total energy: TE} = \text{KE} + \text{PE}$$

$$\text{TE} =$$

$$\text{Velocity: } v =$$

When the Person Is 2 m From the Water (3 m From the Top of the Diving Platform)

$$\text{Total energy: TE} =$$

$$\text{Potential energy: PE} =$$

$$\text{Kinetic energy: KE} =$$

$$\text{Velocity: } v =$$

Vertical Jump Problem

A person with a mass of 50 kg is performing a vertical jump. Their initial *y* velocity is 4.5 m/s. Calculate their energy totals at different phases of the jump.

At the Beginning of the Jump

$$\text{Potential energy: PE} = m\text{*}a_g\text{*}h$$

$$\text{PE} =$$

$$\text{Kinetic energy: KE} = \tfrac{1}{2}\text{*}m\text{*}v^2$$

$$\text{KE} =$$

$$\text{Total energy: TE} = \text{PE} + \text{KE}$$

$$\text{TE} =$$

Initial vertical velocity: 4.5 m/s

At the Apex of the Jump

$$h = \frac{v_y^2}{2*a_g} \quad (h = \text{The maximum height of the jump.})$$

Potential energy: PE = $m\star a_g \star h$

PE =

Kinetic energy: KE = ½ $m\star v^2$

KE =

Total energy: TE = KE + PE

TE =

Velocity: 0 m/s

0.5 m Off the Ground

Let's calculate these variables when the jumper is 0.5 m off the ground, on his or her way up.

Potential energy: PE = $m\star a_g \star h$

PE =

Kinetic energy: Since TE = KE + PE, KE = TE – PE

KE =

Velocity: Since we know kinetic energy, we can use this equation to solve for velocity.

KE = ½$\star m \star v^2$

$v =$

Work

A person applies 800 N of force to move an object 12 m. How much work have they done?

W =

The quadriceps produces 96 Nm of torque to move the lower leg and foot through an angular displacement of 1.70 rad. How much work has the hamstring done?

W =

Power

If a person does 9,200 J of work in 13 s, what is their power output?

P =

If a person applies 350 N of force to move an object at a velocity of 6 m/s, what is their power output in watts?

P =

LABORATORY ACTIVITY 11.1

LABORATORY REPORT

This laboratory report is to be completed outside of the laboratory before the next laboratory meeting.

A person as is jumping off an 8 m high diving platform. Let's assume the person has a mass of 73 kg. What is their potential energy, kinetic energy, total energy, and velocity?

At the Top of the 8 m Diving Platform

$$\text{Potential energy: PE} = m \star a_{g} \star h$$

$$\text{PE} =$$

$$\text{Kinetic energy: KE} = \tfrac{1}{2} \star m \star v^2$$

$$\text{KE} =$$

$$\text{Total energy: TE} = \text{KE} + \text{PE}$$

$$\text{TE} =$$

$$\text{Velocity: } \boldsymbol{v} =$$

When the Person Is 6 m From the Water (2 m From the Top of the Diving Platform)

$$\text{Total energy: TE} =$$

$$\text{Potential energy: PE} =$$

$$\text{Kinetic energy: KE} =$$

$$\text{Velocity:}$$

One person from the laboratory will perform a vertical jump. Your laboratory instructor will record the jump and send you their initial vertical ($\boldsymbol{y}$) velocity. You can use the mass of the person, but to simplify things, we will use a mass of 90 kg.

At the Beginning of the Jump

$$\text{Potential energy: PE} = ma_{g}h$$

$$\text{PE} =$$

$$\text{Kinetic energy: KE} = \tfrac{1}{2}\, mv^2$$

$$\text{KE} =$$

$$\text{Total energy: TE} = \text{PE} + \text{KE}$$

$$\text{TE} =$$

$$\text{Velocity: } 4.5 \text{ m/s}$$

From J. Garner, C. Allen, H. Chander, and A. Knight, *Applied Biomechanics Laboratory Manual.* (Champaign, IL: Human Kinetics, 2023).

At the Apex of the Jump

$$h = \frac{v_y^2}{2 * a_g} \quad (h = \text{ the maximum height of the jump})$$

Potential energy: PE = $ma_g h$

PE =

Kinetic energy: KE = ½*m*v^2

KE =

Total energy: TE = KE + PE

TE =

Velocity: 0 m/s

When the Jumper Is 0.3 m off the Ground

Let's calculate these variables when the jumper is 0.3 m off the ground, on his or her way up.

Potential energy: PE = $ma_g h$

PE =

Kinetic energy: Since TE = KE + PE, KE = TE – PE

KE =

Velocity: Since we know kinetic energy, we can use this equation to solve for velocity:

KE = ½ mv^2

v =

Work

A person applies 300 N of force to move an object 18 m. How much work have they done?

W =

The hamstring produces 106 Nm of torque to move the lower leg and foot through an angular displacement of 1.50 rad. How much work has the hamstring done?

W =

Power

If a person does 6,400 J of work in 16 s, what is their power output?

P =

If a person applies 650 N of force to move an object at a velocity of 8 m/s, what is their power output?

P =

The unit of measurement for power is watts (W).

From J. Garner, C. Allen, H. Chander, and A. Knight, *Applied Biomechanics Laboratory Manual*. (Champaign, IL: Human Kinetics, 2023).

Postural Control and Balance

Objectives

■ Understand the principles of postural control and balance in humans, including the role of the sensory and motor components of the postural control system in maintaining upright erect posture and preventing falling.

■ Learn to assess an individual's balance performance using various balance tests.

■ Understand results from the balance tests and apply to identifying fall risk.

DEFINITIONS

balance—The ability to maintain the center of mass within the base of support. Also known as postural stability (Winter, 1995).

base of support (BOS)—The area bounded by every point of contact that an object or individual uses to make contact with the supporting surface. For humans in an erect bilateral standing position, it is the area bounded posteriorly by the tips of the heels and anteriorly by a line joining the tips of the toes (Levangie & Norkin, 2019) and changes with different static (standing, sitting, lying) and dynamic (walking, running) postures.

center of mass (COM)—The point on a body that moves in the same way that a particle subject to the same external forces would move. It is the point at which all mass acts on the body. For humans, it is also considered as the point where the three midcardinal (midsagittal, midfrontal and midtransverse) planes meet. Anatomically, it is located just anterior to the second sacral vertebra (Rodgers & Cavanagh, 1984).

center of pressure (COP)—A quantity, usually available from a force platform, describing the centroid of the pressure distribution within the BOS. It is also thought of as the point of application of the ground reaction force vector (Rodgers & Cavanagh, 1984).

Postural control is considered to be a complex dynamic interaction of sensory and motor responses in accomplishing the functional tasks by maintaining postural orientation and postural equilibrium (Horak et al., 2006). Postural control can also be defined as the ability to maintain stability of the body and its segments in response to the forces that disturb the body's equilibrium (Levangie & Norkin, 2019). Maintenance of postural equilibrium occurs when all forces acting on the body are balanced so that the body rests in an intended position (static equilibrium) or when a person is able to progress through an intended movement without losing balance (dynamic equilibrium) (Kandel, Schwartz & Jessell, 2021). The postural control mechanism is a result of the sensory systems (visual, vestibular, and somatosensory or proprioceptive) and the motor systems (neuromusculoskeletal) working together with integration from the central nervous system. Degradation of any aspect of the postural control system will result in an abated ability to maintain upright balance and an increased risk of falls and fall-related injuries.

BASIC CONCEPTS OF POSTURAL CONTROL AND BALANCE

To maintain optimal balance and postural stability, the relationship between the COM and BOS must be understood. An object's or an individual's balance and stability depend on the interaction of COM with the BOS following these basic concepts: (1) the larger the area of the BOS, the greater the balance and stability; (2) the closer the COM is to the BOS, the greater the balance and stability; and (3) an object or an individual cannot be perfectly stable, unless the COM is within the BOS.

APPLICATION OF CONCEPTS AND ASSESSMENTS OF BALANCE TO DIFFERENT POPULATIONS

The maintenance of balance is critical under both static and dynamic conditions and is not only important for humans to participate in daily activities of living, but also critical in specific tasks such as competitive sports and occupational tasks. Additionally, falls and fall-related injuries are one of the leading causes of both fatal and nonfatal injuries in various populations such as geriatric, occupational, and certain clinical populations. Moreover, balance training in fall-risk populations can lower the incidence of falls and improve balance performance. Hence, assessments of an individual's balance can provide an understanding of the overall status of the postural control system and can help in the diagnosis, prognosis, rehabilitation, training, and prevention of falls and fall-related injuries.

Basic Assessments of Balance Using Clinical Tests

Assessment of balance in a quick and easy way carries the utmost importance in clinical settings due to the large volume of patients seen with limited time and resources available. Additionally, these tests help keep track of the progression of rehabilitation programs, especially in the absence of sophisticated and expensive balance assessment computerized systems.

Purpose

To assess the balance and postural stability of an individual using clinically relevant balance tests such as Berg's Balance Scale (BBS), the Balance Error Scoring System (BESS), and the Star Excursion Balance Test (SEBT).

Equipment

- Paper
- Pencil or pen
- Stopwatch
- Two standard chairs
- Walkway
- Tape measure
- Soft cushion (AIREX pad)
- Footstool

Berg's Balance Test

Use Berg's Balance Test to complete the scoring from 0 to 4, where 0 indicates the lowest level of function and 4 the highest level of function. A total score is calculated out of 56 maximum possible points, which indicates normal functional balance, while a score of <45 indicates greater risk for falling. Please ask the participant for a history of any previous lower extremity injuries such as ankle sprains and record them, along with identifying dominant and nondominant extremities (adapted from Berg et al., 1992).

1. Sitting to Standing

   Instructions: Please stand up without using your hands for support.

   ( ) 4 able to stand without using hands and stabilize independently

   ( ) 3 able to stand independently using hands

   ( ) 2 able to stand using hands after several tries

   ( ) 1 needs minimal aid to stand or stabilize

   ( ) 0 needs moderate or maximal assistance to stand

2. Standing Unsupported

   Instructions: Please stand for 2 minutes without any support.
   ( ) 4 able to stand safely for 2 minutes
   ( ) 3 able to stand 2 minutes with supervision
   ( ) 2 able to stand 30 seconds unsupported
   ( ) 1 needs several tries to stand 30 seconds unsupported
   ( ) 0 unable to stand 30 seconds unsupported

   If a subject is able to stand 2 minutes unsupported, score full points for sitting unsupported. Proceed to item number 4.

3. Sitting With Back Unsupported but Feet Supported on Floor or on a Stool

   Instructions: Please sit with arms folded for 2 minutes.
   ( ) 4 able to sit safely and securely for 2 minutes
   ( ) 3 able to sit 2 minutes under supervision
   ( ) 2 able to able to sit 30 seconds
   ( ) 1 able to sit 10 seconds
   ( ) 0 unable to sit without support 10 seconds

4. Standing to Sitting

   Instructions: Please sit down.
   ( ) 4 sits safely with minimal use of hands
   ( ) 3 controls descent by using hands
   ( ) 2 uses back of legs against chair to control descent
   ( ) 1 sits independently but has uncontrolled descent
   ( ) 0 needs assistance to sit

5. Transfers

   Instructions: Arrange chairs for pivot transfer. Ask participant to transfer one way toward a seat with armrests and one way toward a seat without armrests.
   ( ) 4 able to transfer safely with minor use of hands
   ( ) 3 able to transfer safely with definite need of hands
   ( ) 2 able to transfer with verbal cuing or supervision
   ( ) 1 needs one person to assist
   ( ) 0 needs two people to assist or supervise to be safe

6. Standing Unsupported With Eyes Closed

   Instructions: Please close your eyes and stand still for 10 seconds.
   ( ) 4 able to stand 10 seconds safely
   ( ) 3 able to stand 10 seconds with supervision
   ( ) 2 able to stand 3 seconds
   ( ) 1 unable to keep eyes closed 3 seconds but stays safely
   ( ) 0 needs help to keep from falling

7. Standing Unsupported With Feet Together

Instructions: Place your feet together and stand without support.

( ) 4 able to place feet together independently and stand 1 minute safely

( ) 3 able to place feet together independently and stand 1 minute with supervision

( ) 2 able to place feet together independently but unable to hold for 30 seconds

( ) 1 needs help to attain position but able to stand 15 seconds, feet together

( ) 0 needs help to attain position and unable to hold for 15 seconds

8. Reaching Forward With Outstretched Arm While Standing

Instructions: Lift arm to 90°. Stretch out your fingers and reach forward as far as you can. (Examiner places a ruler at the end of fingertips when arm is at 90°. The subject's fingers should not touch the ruler while reaching forward. The recorded measure is the distance forward that the fingers reach while the subject is in the most forward lean position. When possible, ask the subject to use both arms when reaching to avoid rotation of the trunk.)

( ) 4 can reach forward confidently 25 cm (10 inches)

( ) 3 can reach forward 12 cm (5 inches)

( ) 2 can reach forward 5 cm (2 inches)

( ) 1 reaches forward but needs supervision

( ) 0 loses balance while trying or requires external support

9. Pick up Object From the Floor From a Standing Position

Instructions: Pick up an object, such as a slipper, which is placed in front of your feet.

( ) 4 able to pick up the slipper safely and easily

( ) 3 able to pick up the slipper but needs supervision

( ) 2 unable to pick up but reaches 2 to 5 cm (1-2 inches) from the slipper and keeps balance independently

( ) 1 unable to pick up the slipper and needs supervision while trying

( ) 0 unable to try or needs assistance to keep from losing balance or falling

10. Turning to Look Behind Over Left and Right Shoulders While Standing

Instructions: Turn to look directly behind you over the left shoulder. Repeat over the right shoulder.

( ) 4 looks behind from both sides and weight shifts well

( ) 3 looks behind one side only; the other side shows less weight shift

( ) 2 turns sideways only but maintains balance

( ) 1 needs supervision when turning

( ) 0 needs assistance to keep from losing balance or falling

11. Turn 360°

Instructions: Turn completely around in a full circle. Pause. Then turn a full circle in the other direction.

( ) 4 able to turn 360° safely in 4 seconds or less

( ) 3 able to turn 360° safely one side only 4 seconds or less

( ) 2 able to turn 360° safely but slowly

( ) 1 needs close supervision or verbal cuing

( ) 0 needs assistance while turning

12. Place Alternate Foot on Step or Stool While Standing Unsupported

Instructions: Place each foot alternately on the footstool. Continue until each foot has contacted the footstool four times.

( ) 4 able to stand independently and safely and complete eight steps in 20 seconds

( ) 3 able to stand independently and complete eight steps in >20 seconds

( ) 2 able to complete four steps without aid with supervision

( ) 1 able to complete >two steps and needs minimal assistance

( ) 0 needs assistance to keep from falling or is unable to try

13. Standing Unsupported With One Foot in Front

Instructions: (demonstrate to the subject) Place one foot directly in front of the other. If you feel that you cannot place your foot directly in front, try to step far enough ahead that the heel of your forward foot is ahead of the toes of the other foot. (To score 3 points, the length of the step should exceed the length of the other foot and the width of the stance should approximate the subject's normal stride width.)

( ) 4 able to place feet tandem independently and hold 30 seconds

( ) 3 able to place one foot ahead independently and hold 30 seconds

( ) 2 able to take a small step independently and hold 30 seconds

( ) 1 needs help to step but can hold 15 seconds

( ) 0 loses balance while stepping or standing

14. Standing on One Leg

Instructions: Stand on one leg as long as you can without any support.

( ) 4 able to lift leg independently and hold >10 seconds

( ) 3 able to lift leg independently and hold 5 to 10 seconds

( ) 2 able to lift leg independently and hold ≥3 seconds

( ) 1 tries to lift leg, is unable to hold 3 seconds, but remains standing independently

( ) 0 unable to try or needs assistance to prevent fall

_____ **total score (maximum = 56)**

Question Set 12.1 (BBS)

1. Based on the total score, make interpretations of the status of functional balance in the assessed individuals.
2. Were there any differences in individuals with and without previous history of lower extremity injuries?
3. What is the risk of falling based on the observed score, and how do they compare to the normative scores?

Balance Error Scoring System

The Balance Error Scoring System (BESS) consists of standing with the eyes closed on two surface conditions in three stance positions that includes (1) double-legged stance with hands on hips with feet together, (2) single-legged stance with hands on hips and standing on the nondominant leg, and (3) a tandem stance with hands on hips and the nondominant foot behind the dominant foot. The first surface is a flat-firm surface, and the second is performed on a foam or cushion surface (AIREX balance pad) to create a total of six testing conditions with each condition being tested for 20 seconds (adapted from Bell et al., 2011).

Step 1: Explain the description of each of the conditions of BESS to the participant.

Step 2: Start with the three stance conditions on the firm surface and then progress to the foam condition.

Step 3: During the 20-second trials, the number of errors is calculated by adding one error point for each error. Errors and their types are mentioned after these steps. Use the BESS scorecard to complete the BESS.

Step 4: Please ask for participant history of any previous lower extremity injuries such as ankle sprains to record it, along with identifying the dominant and nondominant extremities.

BESS—Types of Errors

The maximum total number of errors for any single condition is 10.

- Hands lifted off the hips
- Opening eyes
- Step, stumble, loss of balance, or fall
- Moving the hip >30° abduction
- Lifting the forefoot or heel from the original position
- Failing to return to the test position in less than 5 seconds

BESS Scorecard—Number of Errors

Stance conditions	Firm surface	Foam surface
Double-legged stance (feet together)		
Single-legged stance (nondominant leg)		
Tandem stance (nondominant leg behind dominant leg)		
BESS total error score		

Question Set 12.1 BESS

1. Based on the total score, make interpretations of the status of functional balance in the assessed individuals.

2. Were there any differences in individuals with and without a previous history of lower extremity injuries?

3. What is the risk of falling based on the observed score, and how do they compare to the normative scores?

Star Excursion Balance Test

The Star Excursion Balance Test (SEBT) is a dynamic test of balance very commonly used in athletic populations, especially when screening for lower extremity injuries and during rehabilitation after injuries (figure 12.1). The test involves standing on one leg at a time on the center of four strips of athletic tape that are 6 ft long placed on the floor crossing each other in a star-shaped pattern so that each of the tape lines are at a 45° angle with each other to have eight different directions (anterior, anteromedial, medial, posteromedial, posterior, posterolateral, lateral, and anterolateral). Each of the eight directions of the tape is marked with incremental marks from the center (cm or in.) so it is easy to observe and record the reaching distance.

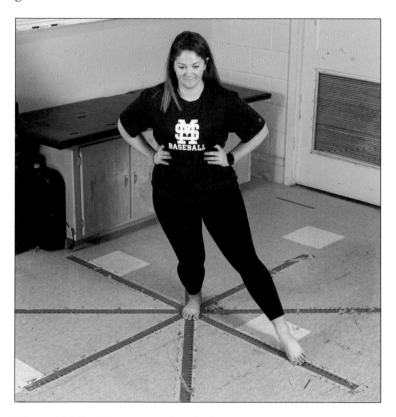

Figure 12.1   Star excursion balance test.

Step 1:   Explain the SEBT to the participant.

Step 2:   Start with one leg of the participant placed in the center of the star pattern and instruct the participant to reach as far as possible with the contralateral leg in each of the 8 directions, without losing balance on the stance leg and without bearing too much weight on the reaching leg. Ensure that the reaching leg must only do a gentle tap on the maximum possible distance on the tape, rather than shifting weight on to the reaching leg.

Step 3:   Use the table after step 4 to record reaching distance.

Step 4:   Ask for participant history of any previous lower extremity injuries such as ankle sprains to record it, along with identifying dominant and nondominant extremities.

SEBT

Reach directions	Reach distance—left leg	Reach distance—right leg
Anterior		
Anteromedial		
Medial		
Posteromedial		
Posterior		
Posterolateral		
Lateral		
Anterolateral		

Question Set 12.1 SEBT

1. Based on the reaching distances in each leg, make interpretations of the status of functional balance in the assessed individuals.

2. Are there any differences in individuals with and without previous history of lower extremity injuries?

3. Are there any differences between dominant and nondominant extremities?

Assessments of Balance Using Force Platforms and Balance Systems

Beyond clinical paper-based and observation balance tests, more objective postural control data are measured using modern technology relying on kinematic and kinetic data, especially in a research laboratory setting. Various computerized balance systems such as force platforms to dedicated balance systems such as NeuroCom Equitest and Biodex Balance machines are used. Cost-effective and easy-to-use balance plate systems such as the BTrackS balance plates have been developed. The advantage of these sophisticated balance assessment systems includes the ability to manipulate sensory feedback and have more detailed analyses of postural control parameters using variables such as COP derived from the force platforms.

Purpose

The purpose of this lab activity is to assess balance with the manipulation of sensory inputs to maintain balance. The modified clinical test of sensory integration in balance (mCTSIB) consists of four conditions in bilateral stance: (1) eyes open standing on firm surface; (2) eyes closed on firm surface; (3) eyes open on foam surface; and (4) eyes closed on foam surface (figure 12.2). In condition 1, all three sensory systems (visual, vestibular, and somatosensory or proprioceptive) are available. In condition 2, only vestibular and somatosensory or proprioceptive are available absent vision. In condition 3, the somatosensory or proprioceptive system is compromised, and in condition 4, in addition to the compromised somatosensory or proprioceptive system, visual feedback is absent. The mCTSIB can also be conducted on instrumented devices such as force platforms.

Procedures

Explain the four conditions to the participant and instruct them to stand as still as possible in each of the testing conditions. Instruct the participant with eyes open or closed and standing on a firm surface or foam surface accordingly for 30 seconds for three trials. If the participant is able to perform the full 30 seconds without losing balance, you can limit the trials to one. If not, an average of the three trials are taken. The time spent in each trial of each condition is assessed. Begin the timing at the beginning of each trial, and a trial is over at the end of a successful 30 s interval or when the participant opens their eyes, raises their arms, or loses their balance. When performing the assessment with an instrumented force plate, postural sway variables can be calculated using the systems software, or the COP trajectories can be exported and calculated after data collection. Use the table that follows to complete the mCTSIB assessment. Please ask for participant history of any previous lower extremity injuries such as ankle sprains and record them, along with identifying the dominant and nondominant extremities.

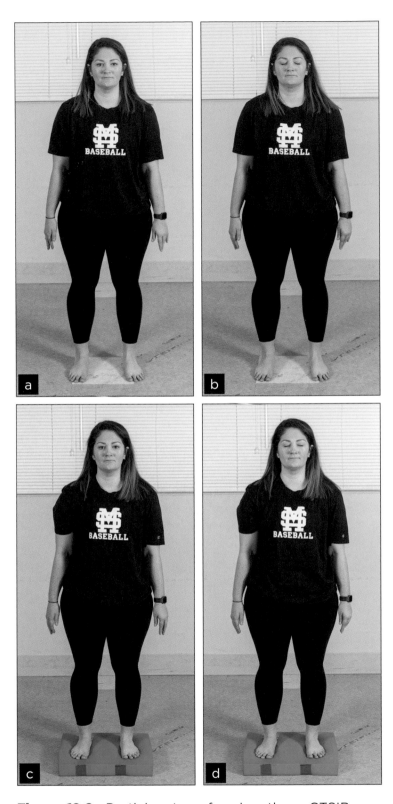

Figure 12.2 Participant performing the mCTSIB assessment on a (*a-b*) firm surface with the eyes open and closed, and on a (*c-d*) foam surface with the eyes open and closed.

mCTSIB

Condition	Trial 1	Trial 2	Trial 3
Eyes open, firm surface			
Eyes closed, firm surface			
Eyes open, foam surface			
Eyes closed, foam surface			

Question Set 12.2

1. Based on the reaching distances in each leg, make interpretations of the status of functional balance in the assessed individuals.

2. Were there any differences in individuals with and without a previous history of lower extremity injuries?

3. What is the risk of falling based on the observed score, and how does it compare to the normative scores?

Distinguishing Postural Responses

Compensatory postural responses are reactive responses that work to regain equilibrium following a postural perturbation depending on feedback from sensory systems. On the contrary, proactive responses while anticipating a postural perturbation with a feet-forward mechanism are called anticipatory postural responses.

This laboratory activity will explore the use of compensatory and anticipatory postural adjustments in an object-holding task.

Equipment

- Paper
- Pen or pencil
- Stadiometer or a vertically oriented tape measure
- Object such as a sandbag, an ankle weight, or a heavy textbook that is around 10 lb (44.5 N; or any similar mass).

Step 1: Choose a student volunteer as the participant.

Step 2: Instruct the participant to stand next to a stadiometer, stretching one of their arms to perform 90° of shoulder flexion with the elbow straight and the palm facing up.

Step 3: Place a 10 lb (44.5 N) object on the participant's palm and ask them to maintain the same position.

Step 4: Make a note of the height on the stadiometer at the level of the fingers of the stretched, object-holding arm.

Step 5: Ask the participant to close their eyes for the first condition. Without any warning and at a random time interval, remove the object quickly without touching the participant's hand. Note the movement of the arm across the stadiometer and measure in centimeters of the displacement of the arm from the original position.

Step 6: For the next condition, instruct the participant to assume the same position and place the same object on their palm.

Step 7: Ask the participant to keep their eyes opened for this condition, and while counting loudly, "3, 2, 1," lift the object quickly in the same manner as earlier.

Step 8: Notice and measure the displacement of the arm and compare with the previous eyes-open condition. This can also be performed using a digital camera and using software such as Dartfish or MaxTRAQ for angular measurements of the shoulder joint movement.

Question Set 12.3

1. What was the shoulder movement observed in each of the conditions?
2. How much did the arm (cm) or the shoulder joint (degrees) move in each of the conditions? Which condition had a greater linear or angular displacement?
3. Why was one condition different from the other? Provide rationale for differences between conditions.
4. Identify evidence of compensatory postural responses and anticipatory postural responses from the two conditions.

Gait and Locomotion

Objectives

- Understand the principles of gait and locomotion.
- Learn gait terminology regarding temporal and spatial parameters as well as concepts of human gait.
- Learn to perform lab-based gait assessments and calculate gait variables in different activities.

DEFINITIONS

gait cycle—The sequence of lower extremity events, from initial contact of one extremity onto the supporting surface to the next subsequent initial contact of the same extremity onto the supporting surface (Enoka, 2015; Winter, 1995).

gait cycle phases—Division of a gait cycle into two parts, each with its own subdivisions. The stance phase (60% of the gait cycle) occurs when the foot of the reference lower extremity is in contact with the supporting surface, and the swing phase (40% of the gait cycle) occurs when the foot is not in contact with the supporting surface. The stance phase is divided into initial contact, foot flat, midstance, heel-off, and toe-off while the swing phase is divided into early swing, midswing, and late swing (Levangie & Norkin, 2019).

Analysis of gait is an excellent measure of the body's central and peripheral nervous system, sensory and motor systems, musculoskeletal system, and even the cardiovascular and respiratory systems. Understanding normal gait is vital, as gait deviations can be easily identified and can be indicative of pathologies of the aforementioned systems. Human gait and locomotion are described as a translatory progression of the body as a whole, accomplished by coordinated angular movements of the body segments.

Laboratory activity 13.1 builds on top of the linear kinematics laboratory activity (laboratory 4) that involved calculation of running kinematic variables such as displacement, velocity, and acceleration, using a running activity. In this laboratory activity, a similar running activity will be used to calculate gait parameters focusing on some of the most basic descriptors of running performance—speed, step length, step time, and step rate (step frequency). Gait parameters will be investigated during two different types of running activities. The first type (A) focuses on distance running kinematics and the second (B) on sprinting kinematics. The purposes of this experiment are (1) to describe the motion of an athlete performing a 25 m run and (2) to demonstrate the relationships that exist between the quantities used to describe the motion (in a 50 m run).

TEMPORAL AND SPATIAL PARAMETERS OF GAIT

The following selected temporal and spatial parameters of gait will be used in this lab.

- **Step**—One half of a complete stride (e.g., right foot contact to left foot contact).
- **Step length (SL)**—The distance traveled per step.
- **Step rate (SR)**—The rate at which steps are taken (i.e., number of steps per unit of

time); inverse of step time. Also known as step frequency.

- **Step time (ST)**—The time required to complete one step.
- **Stride**—The basic unit of motion for gait reflecting one complete cycle of motion; the motion occurring between successive contacts of the same foot (e.g., right-foot contact to next right-foot contact).

Calculation for average running speed. S = speed, SL = step length, SR = step rate, t = time.

$$\bar{s} = \ell/\Delta t$$

average running speed = (avg. step length)/ (avg. step time)

$$\bar{s} = \overline{SL}/\overline{ST}$$

average running speed = avg. step length × avg. step rate

$$\bar{s} = \overline{SL} \times \overline{ST}$$

Running Gait Analysis

Equipment

- Paper
- Pencil or pen
- Calculator
- Stopwatches (two sets)
- Tape measure
- Cones
- Whistle
- Individual laboratory report
- Whiteboard or other writing surface

Part 1: Calculation of Step Length, Step Rate, and Speed During a 25 m Run Course

Step 1:   Have the participant run through the course of 25 m four times at four different speeds (slow, medium, fast, and all out). The subject should try to maintain a constant speed through the 25 m course; therefore, they will begin approximately 10 m behind the starting line (figure 13.1).

Step 2:   Using two sets of stopwatches, record two different times for the runner: (1) the time to cover 25 m and (2) the time to cover a given number of steps (e.g., 10 steps). Note: The number of complete steps is always one less than the number of foot strikes. Therefore, begin your count (and your stopwatches) with step 0 rather than step 1. This will give you the correct number of steps. Average speed is computed by dividing the total distance by the total time. Average step rate is computed by dividing the

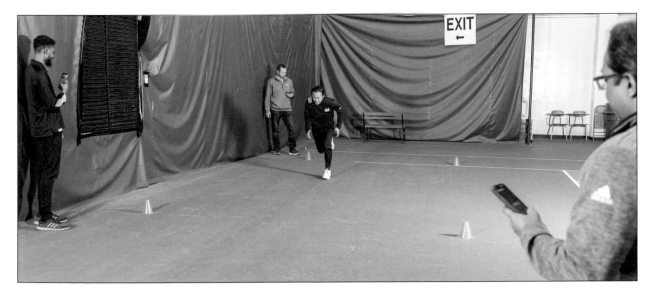

Figure 13.1   Example setup of a 25 m run course.

set number of steps by the time it takes to complete those steps. Average step length is computed by dividing the average speed by the average step rate.

Step 3: Record the results in table 13.1 on the individual laboratory report.

This lab is accompanied by a video demonstration in HK*Propel*.

Part 2: Calculation of Velocity and Acceleration Profiles

Step 1: Have the participant stand at the starting line of a 50 m run course. Note: A different participant should be used for this part.

Step 2: Position the starter at the starting line and place one or two timers at each of the remaining lines (i.e., 10 m, 20 m, 30 m, 40 m, and finish line at 50 m).

Step 3: Have the starter signal the timers to synchronously start their watches as the starting signal is given to the subject.

Step 4: As the torso of the subject reaches the 10 m line, the timers standing opposite that line stop their watches.

Step 5: Repeat the process at the 20 m line, the 30 m line, the 40 m line, and the finish line at 50 m. In effect, we are taking splits at 10 m intervals.

Step 6: Record the times on a whiteboard.

Step 7: Repeat this process two more times for a total of three trials.

Step 8: Average the results among the three trials. Note: Between trials, the timers should move to a different line to minimize the effect of any one person's timing errors on the results. The purpose of averaging across trials is to reduce error.

Step 9: Record the results in table 13.2 on the individual laboratory report.

Question Set 13.1

1. Use the data collected in part 1 to complete table 13.1. Note: SL stands for step length and SR stands for step rate.

2. From the data collected in part 2, complete table 13.2.

3. Calculate the average velocity over each 10 m interval (i.e., 0-10 m, 10-20 m, etc.). Use Microsoft Excel and plot these values in the form of a histogram (bar graph) with velocities (y-axis) plotted as a function of position (x-axis). In addition, calculate the average velocity over the entire 50 m and indicate this value by a dotted line across the entire histogram. Show all your calculations on a separate page and complete table 13.3.

4. After examining the results, what can you report about the performance of the participant in part 2? Did they continue to speed up through the entire run or slow down a bit at the end? Where was peak velocity reached (in terms of both position and time)?

INDIVIDUAL LABORATORY REPORT

Participant name or ID number: _____ Date: _____

Tester: _____ Time: _____

Participant age: _____ Height: _____ Weight: _____ Sex: _____

Table 13.1 Raw Data and Results for Part 1

Trial	Distance (m)	Time 1 (s)	Avg. speed (m/s)	No. of steps	Avg. SR (steps/s)	Avg. SL (m/step)
1. Slow	25					
2. Medium	25					
3. Fast	25					
4. All out	25					

Table 13.2 Raw Data and Computed Mean Split Times for Part 2

SPLIT TIMES (S)					
0 m	10 m	20 m	30 m	40 m	50 m
3.33					

Table 13.3 Computes Average Velocities at Each Interval in Part 2

Variable	INTERVAL					
	0-10 m	10-20 m	20-30 m	30-40m	40 50 m	50 m
d (m)	10	10	10	10	10	50
t (s)						
$\bar{v}$ (m/s)						

Treadmill or Overground Gait Analyses

In a laboratory setting, walking on a treadmill is very commonly used and has been compared to overground walking, especially when analyzing gait for an extended duration and at a controlled speed. Additionally, running on a treadmill still allows the researcher to analyze the running gait with the use of sophisticated instruments such as a motion-capture system and instrumented force plates embedded in the treadmill. Regardless of the equipment used, treadmill gait has the advantage of allowing the gait analysis to be controlled by the researcher.

Purpose

To perform gait analyses and investigate gait parameters while walking on a treadmill at different speeds.

Equipment and Supplies Needed

Based on the availability, a 2D digital camera and biomechanical video analysis software such Dartfish, MaxTRAQ, smartphones with motion-analyses applications, instrumented treadmills, or a 3D motion-capture system can be used.

Procedures

The procedures for this laboratory activity can be modified based on the equipment available. The goal of this laboratory activity is to analyze gait at different speeds of walking (such as 2 mph, 3 mph, and 4 mph [3.2, 4.8, and 6.4 kph, respectively]). If a treadmill is not available, you can still use 2D digital cameras with biomechanical software, smartphones with motion-analysis applications, a 3D motion-capture system, and force plates (portable or embedded in a walkway) for overground gait analyses in different speeds, either individually using one piece of equipment or collectively using some or all the available equipment.

Here are a few guidelines to follow when collecting data using different equipment.

- If using 2D digital camera and video motion-analysis software, use sagittal plane analysis (keeping the camera on the lateral side of the participant). You can also choose to add another camera for frontal plane analyses (usually posterior to the participant to avoid treadmill obstruction of view). Make sure the joint centers such as the ankle joint, knee joint, and hip joint are marked with reflective or contrast tape or marker, to ease identifying joint segments.

- If you are using a 3D motion-capture system, please follow the procedures of the type of the system and software used, such as Vicon, Motion Monitor, Motion Analysis, Qualisys, etc. Depending on the system used, you may be using a lower body or upper body plug-in gait model with reflective markers or marker clusters. Use tight-fitting athletic compression clothing with reflective markers or marker clusters for better marker tracking and avoid anything reflective on the garments other than the markers themselves to avoid errors in the motion-capture system.

- If you are using a force plate embedded in the ground on a walkway, ensure clean foot strikes onto the force plates and that the stance phase occurs with the entire foot on the force plate.
- Gait variables usually analyzed are joint kinematics and kinetics and ground reaction forces. An electromyography system can also be added to analyze muscle activity during gait.

Question Set 13.2

Depending upon the systems and equipment used:

1. How did lower extremity joint kinematics, kinetics, and stance phase or ground reaction phase change with changing speeds?
2. Graph these calculated variables using Microsoft Excel or any motion-capture software for one gait cycle, for each speed.
3. In the graphs, identify the all the subphases of the stance and swing phase of the gait cycle. How do these gait cycle phases change with changing speed?

BIBLIOGRAPHY

Laboratory 1

Enoka, R.M. (2015). *Neuromechanics of human movement* (5th ed.). Human Kinetics.

Floyd, R.T., & Thompson, C. (2020). *Manual of structural kinesiology* (21st ed.). McGraw Hill.

Levangie, P.K., & Norkin, C.C. (2019). *Joint structure and function: A comprehensive analysis* (6th ed.). F.A. Davis.

Laboratory 2

Dempster, W.T. (1955). *Space requirements of the seated operator, geometrical, kinematic, and mechanical aspects of the body with special reference to the limbs.* Michigan State University.

De Leva, P. (1996). Adjustments to Zatsiorsky-Seluyanov's segment inertia parameters. *Journal of biomechanics, 29*(9), 1223-1230.

Levangie, P.K., & Norkin, C.C. (2019). *Joint structure and function: A comprehensive analysis.* (6th ed.). F.A. Davis.

Magee, D.J., & Manske, R.C. (2020). *Orthopedic physical assessment* (7th ed.). Elsevier.

Norkin, C.C., & White, D.J. (2016). *Measurement of joint motion: A guide to goniometry* (5th ed.). F.A. Davis.

Zatsiorsky, V. M. (1990). Methods of determing mass-inertial characteristics of human body segments. *Contemporasy Problems of Biomechnics.*

Laboratory 5

Burkett, B. (2019). *Applied sport mechanics.* Human Kinetics.

Enoka, R.M. (2015). *Neuromechanics of human movement.* Human Kinetics.

Flanagan, S.P. (2019). *Biomechanics: A case-based approach.* Jones & Bartlett Learning.

Winter, D.A. (2009). *Biomechanics and motor control of human movement.* John Wiley and Sons, Inc.

Laboratory 6

Burkett, B. (2019). *Applied sport mechanics.* Human Kinetics.

Enoka, R.M. (2015). *Neuromechanics of human movement.* Human Kinetics.

Flanagan, S.P. (2019). *Biomechanics: A case-based approach.* Jones & Bartlett Learning.

Winter, D.A. (2009). *Biomechanics and motor control of human movement.* John Wiley and Sons, Inc.

Laboratory 7

Attwells, R.L., Birrell, S.A., Hooper, R.H., & Mansfield, N.J. (2006). Influence of carrying heavy loads on soldiers' posture, movements and gait. *Ergonomics, 49*(14), 1527-1537.

Birrell, S.A., & Haslam, R.A. (2009). The effect of military load carriage on 3-D lower limb kinematics and spatiotemporal parameters. *Ergonomics, 52*(10), 1298-1304.

Birrell, S.A., & Haslam, R.A. (2010). The effect of load distribution within military load carriage systems on the kinetics of human gait. *Applied ergonomics, 41*(4), 585-590.

Chander, H., Kodithuwakku Arachchige, S.N.K., Wilson, S.J., Knight, A.C., Burch, R.F.V., Carruth, D.W., Wade, C., & Garner, J.C. (2020 in press). Impact of military footwear type and load carriage on slip initiation biomechanics. *International Journal of Human Factors and Ergonomics.*

David, G.C. (2005). Ergonomic methods for assessing exposure to risk factors for work-related musculoskeletal disorders. *Occupational Medicine, 55*(3), 190-199.

Escamilla, R.F., Fleisig, G.S., DeRenne, C., Taylor, M., Moorman, C.T., Imamura, R. & Andrews, J.R. (2009). A comparison of age level on baseball hitting kinematics. *Journal of Applied Biomechanics, 25,* 210-218.

Fleisig, G.S., Barrentine, S.W., Zheng, N., Escamilla, R.F., & Andrews, J.R. (1999). Kinematic and kinetic comparison of baseball pitching among various levels of development. *Journal of Biomechanics, 32,* 1371-1375.

Fry, A.C., Smith, J.C., & Schilling, B.K. (2003). Effect of knee position on hip and knee torque during the barbell squat. *The Journal of Strength and Conditioning Research, 17*(4), 629-633.

Hertel, J. (2019). An updated model of chronic ankle instability. *Journal of Athletic Training, 54*(6), 572-588.

Herzog, M.M., Kerr, Z.Y., Marshall, S.W., & Wikstrom, E.A. (2019). Epidemiology of ankle sprains and chronic ankle instability. *Journal of Athletic Training, 54*(6), 603-610.

Konradsen, L., Voigt, M., & Hojsgaard, C. (1997). Ankle inversion injuries: The role of the dynamic defense mechanism. *American Journal of Sports Medicine, 25*(1), 54-58.

Kumar, S. (Ed.). (2007). *Biomechanics in ergonomics* (2nd ed.). CRC Press.

Li, Y., Ko, J., Zhang, S., Brown, C.N., & Simpson, K.J. (2019). Biomechanics of ankle giving way: A case report of accidental ankle giving way during the drop landing test. *Journal of Sport and Health Science, 8*(5), 494-502.

List, R., Gulay, T., Stoop, M., & Lorenzetti, S. (2013). Kinematics of the trunk and the lower extremities during restricted and unrestricted squats. *The Journal of Strength and Conditioning Research, 27*(6), 1529-1538.

Majumdar, D., Pal, M.S., & Majumdar, D. (2010). Effects of military load carriage on kinematics of gait. *Ergonomics, 53*(6), 782-791.

Papadopoulos, E., Nicolopoulos, C., Anderson, E., Curran, M., & Athanasopoulos, S. (2005). The role of ankle bracing in injury prevention, athletic performance and neuromuscular control: A review of the literature. *The Foot, 15*(1), 1-6.

Punnett, L., & Wegman, D.H. (2004). Work-related musculoskeletal disorders: The epidemiologic evidence and the debate. *Journal of Electromyography and Kinesiology, 14*(1), 13-23.

Putnam, C.A. (1983). Sequential motions of body segments in striking and throwing skills: Description and explanations. *Journal of Biomechanics, 26*(Suppl), 125-135.

Whitting, J.W., Meir, R.A., Crowley-McHattan, Z.J., & Holding, R.C. (2016). Influence of footwear type on barbell back squat using 50, 70, and 90% of one repetition maximum: A biomechanical analysis. *The Journal of Strength and Conditioning Research, 30*(4), 1085-1092.

Laboratory 8

Chavda, S., Bromley, T., Jarvis, P., Williams, S., Bishop, C., Turner, A.N., Lake, J.P., Mundy, P.D. (2018). Force-time characteristics of the countermovement jump: Analyzing the curve in Excel. *Strength & Conditioning Journal, 40*, 67-77.

Cormie, P., McGuigan, M.R., & Newton, R.U. (2010a). Adaptations in athletic performance after ballistic power versus strength training. *Medicine & Science in Sports & Exercise, 42*, 1582-1598.

Cormie, P., McGuigan, M.R., & Newton, R.U. (2010b). Influence of strength on magnitude and mechanisms of adaptation to power training. *Medicine & Science in Sports & Exercise, 42*, 1566-1581.

Garhammer, J., & Gregor, R. (1992). Propulsion forces as a function of intensity for weightlifting and vertical jumping. *Journal of Applied Sport Science Research, 6*, 129-134.

Pontillo, M., Hines, S., Sennett, B. (2020). Prediction of lower extremity injuries from vertical jump kinetic data in collegiate athletes. *Journal of Orthopaedic and Sports Physical Therapy, 50*, CSM30.

Laboratory 9

Aagaard, P., Simonsen, E.B., Andersen, J.L., Magnusson, P., & Dyhre-Poulsen, P. (2002). Increased rate of force development and neural drive of human skeletal muscle following resistance training. *Journal of Applied Physiology, 93*, 1318-1326.

Chavda, S., Bromley, T., Jarvis, P., Williams, S., Bishop, C., Turner, A.N., Lake, J.P., Mundy, P.D. (2018). Force-time characteristics of the countermovement jump: Analyzing the curve in Excel. *Strength & Conditioning Journal, 40*, 67-77.

Kirby, T.J., McBride, J.M., Haines, T.L., & Dayne, A.M. (2011). Relative net vertical impulse determines jumping performance. *Journal of Applied Biomechanics, 27*, 207-214.

Laffaye, G., & Wagner, P. (2013). Eccentric rate of force development determines jumping performance. *Computer Methods in Biomechanics and Biomedical Engineering, 16,* 82-83.

Winter, E.M. (2005). Jumping: Power or impulse? *Medicine and Science in Sports and Exercise, 37,* 523.

Laboratory 10

Burkett, B. (2019). *Applied sport mechanics.* Human Kinetics.

Enoka, R.M. (2015). *Neuromechanics of human movement.* Human Kinetics.

Flanagan, S.P. (2019). *Biomechanics: A case-based approach.* Jones & Bartlett Learning.

Winter, D.A. (2009). *Biomechanics and motor control of human movement.* John Wiley and Sons, Inc.

Laboratory 11

Burkett, B. (2019). *Applied sport mechanics.* Human Kinetics.

Enoka, R.M. (2015). *Neuromechanics of human movement.* Human Kinetics.

Flanagan, S.P. (2019). *Biomechanics: A case-based approach.* Jones & Bartlett Learning.

Winter, D.A. (2009). *Biomechanics and motor control of human movement.* John Wiley and Sons, Inc.

Laboratory 12

Bell, D.R., Guskiewicz, K.M., Clark, M.A., & Padua, D.A. (2011). Systematic review of the balance error scoring system. *Sports Health, 3*(3), 287-295.

Berg, K., Wood-Dauphinee, S, Williams, J.I., & Maki, B. (1992). Measuring balance in the elderly: Validation of an instrument. *Canadian Journal of Public Health, 2*(July/August supplement), S7-S11.

Enoka, R.M. (2015). *Neuromechanics of human movement* (5th ed.). Human Kinetics.

Horak, F.B. (2006). Postural orientation and equilibrium: What do we need to know about neural control of balance to prevent falls? *Age and Ageing, 35*(suppl 2), ii7-ii11.

Kandel, E.R., Schwartz, J.H., Jessell, T.M., Siegelbaum, S., Hudspeth, A.J., & Mack, S. (Eds.). (2021). *Principles of neural science* (6th ed.). McGraw-Hill.

Levangie, P.K., & Norkin, C.C. (2019). *Joint structure and function: A comprehensive analysis* (6th ed.). F.A. Davis.

Rodgers, M.M., & Cavanagh, P.R. (1984). Glossary of biomechanical terms, concepts, and units. *Physical Therapy, 64*(12), 1886-1902.

Winter, D.A. (1995). Human balance and posture control during standing and walking. *Gait & Posture, 3*(4), 193-214.

Laboratory 13

Enoka, R.M. (2015). *Neuromechanics of human movement* (5th ed.). Human Kinetics.

Levangie, P.K., & Norkin, C.C. (2019). *Joint structure and function: A comprehensive analysis* (6th ed.). F.A. Davis.

Winter, D.A. (1995). Human balance and posture control during standing and walking. *Gait & posture, 3*(4), 193-214.

ABOUT THE AUTHORS

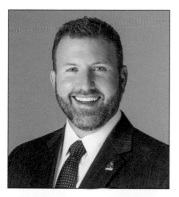

John C. Garner, PhD, CSCS★D, currently serves as the dean of the College of Health and Human Services and a professor of exercise science within the department of kinesiology and health promotion at Troy University. Dr. Garner has written over 250 peer-reviewed research publications, conference proceedings, and presentations, with nearly $2 million in research funding. His research focuses on the biomechanics of human movement in work and sport settings. He holds a Certified Strength and Conditioning Specialist with Distinction (CSCS★D) designation from the National Strength and Conditioning Association. He earned his PhD in biomechanics from Auburn University in 2008.

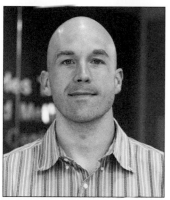

Charles R. Allen, PhD, CSCS★D, TSAC-F, USAW-L1, is an assistant professor in the exercise science program at Florida Southern College. Previously, Dr. Allen served as a fitness professional in the collegiate recreational setting. His research interests center around improving human performance in sport, exercise, and activities of daily living. Allen has written 45 peer-reviewed research publications, conference proceedings, and presentations. He holds the Certified Strength and Conditioning Specialist (CSCS) and Tactical Strength and Conditioning Facilitator (TSAC-F) designations from the National Strength and Conditioning Association. Dr. Allen earned his PhD in kinesiology from the University of Mississippi in 2015.

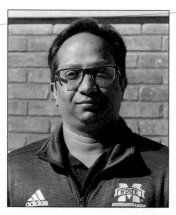

Harish Chander, PhD, is an associate professor of biomechanics and the codirector of the Neuromechanics Laboratory in the department of kinesiology at Mississippi State University, where he teaches and conducts research in biomechanics and neuromechanics. He also serves as the chair for the academic culture committee in the department of kinesiology and as a member of the faculty council in the College of Education. Dr. Chander has written over 237 peer-reviewed research publications, conference proceedings, and presentations. His research centers on the application of principles of biomechanics and neuromechanics to human performance, injury prevention, and safety promotion. He earned his PhD in biomechanics and neuromechanics from the University of Mississippi in 2014.

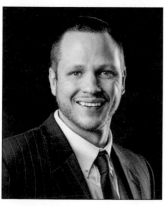

Adam C. Knight, PhD, ATC, CSCS, is a professor of biomechanics and the codirector of the Neuromechanics Laboratory in the department of kinesiology at Mississippi State University, where he also serves as the graduate program coordinator for the department. He has written over 150 peer-reviewed research publications, conference proceedings, and presentations. His research interests include sport biomechanics and the biomechanical implication of chronic ankle instability (CAI). Dr. Knight is a BOC-certified athletic trainer and a member of the National Athletic Trainers' Association and the American Society of Biomechanics. He holds the Certified Strength and Conditioning Specialist (CSCS) designation from the National Strength and Conditioning Association. Knight earned his PhD in biomechanics from Auburn University in 2009.

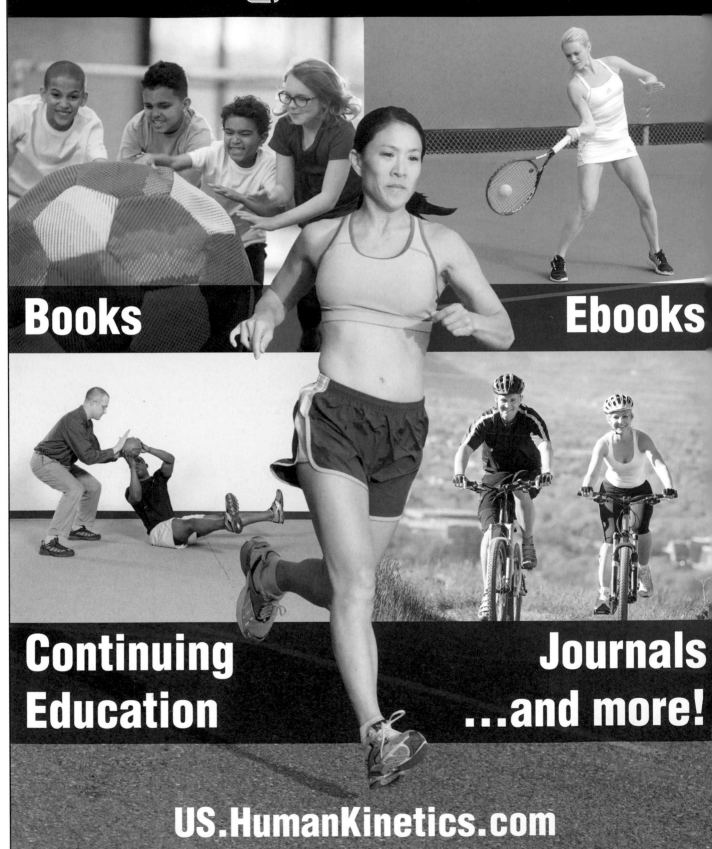